DEVELOPING HEALTHCARE SKILLS THROUGH
SIMULATION

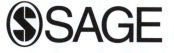

DEVELOPING HEALTHCARE SKILLS THROUGH

SIMULATION

EDITED BY

MATTHEW ALDRIDGE & STEPHEN WANLESS

SAGE

Los Angeles | London | New Delhi
Singapore | Washington DC

First published 2012

Reprinted 2012

SAGE Publications Ltd
1 Oliver's Yard
55 City Road
London EC1Y 1SP

SAGE Publications Inc.
2455 Teller Road
Thousand Oaks, California 91320

SAGE Publications India Pvt Ltd
B 1/I 1 Mohan Cooperative Industrial Area
Mathura Road
New Delhi 110 044

SAGE Publications Asia-Pacific Pte Ltd
3 Church Street
#10-04 Samsung Hub
Singapore 049483

Library of Congress Control Number: 2011936656

British Library Cataloguing in Publication data

A catalogue record for this book is available from the British Library

ISBN 978-1-4462-0124-4
ISBN 978-1-4462-0125-1 (pbk)

Typeset by C&M Digitals (P) Ltd, Chennai, India
Printed and bound by CPI Group (UK) Ltd, Croydon, CR0 4YY
Printed on paper from sustainable resources

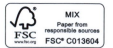

CONTENTS

FOREWORD

It is a pleasure to be invited to prepare a foreword for this publication, not least because the task prompts me to reflect upon where the simulation journey has taken us here at my own institution. As Director of Learning and Teaching at a large and diverse university my main focus is naturally on the student experience.

Our own journey and decision to invest in the development of a simulation centre involved the clear purpose of enhancing our relationship both with healthcare employers and, importantly, with students. Although aware of the growing use of simulation in medical education and its gradual emergence into education for the nursing profession, we had a specific trigger. At the International Council of Nurses Congress in Taiwan in 2005, we witnessed a hugely compelling presentation from three academics from the School of Nursing at University of Pittsburgh.[1] The impact of this presentation did not relate to impressive equipment or indeed to the fidelity of the simulation, but rather to the educational message. The presenters articulated the importance of effective curriculum design and spoke not only of student competence in skills that could be transferred to the clinical environment, but also of student confidence and development of team work skills. On a subsequent visit to Pittsburgh, colleagues and I observed learning activities that placed peer support – senior students working with freshmen, for example – and debrief and feed forward at the centre of educational processes.

For us the message was clear. Investment in facilities would be valuable, but only if accompanied by real attention to curriculum design and recognition that proper and effective use of such opportunities would lead to the development of a much more personalised learning experience for our students. We had an early opportunity when involved in a Nursing and Midwifery Council pilot project 'Simulation and Practice Learning' in 2006. This pilot, run across 13 universities, afforded us and many others an early opportunity to see the profound impact on students and educators of the use of properly designed simulation sessions. We found that shared apprehension quickly turned to enthusiasm, communication between educators and students was enhanced and the potential was obvious. In many ways this relates to the personalisation of learning and empowerment of students in a safe environment. Of particular value is the opportunity for students to revisit their skills development, take active responsibility for their learning and with effective scaffolding of a variety of learning approaches better to relate knowledge to practical situations.

---

1 Burns, H.K., Hoffman, R.L. and O'Donnell, J.M. (2005) 'Enhancing nursing knowledge acquisition through an innovative curricular approach using high fidelity human simulation' International Council of Nursing Annual Conference. Nursing on the Move: Knowledge, Innovation and Vitality, May 2005, Taipei, Taiwan.

I firmly believe that this publication will be invaluable to many as they seek to make judgements about how to incorporate simulation in their work and seek ideas for design of simulation sessions. Such an understanding of the educational basis for the use of simulation, followed by the use of effective design of individual learning episodes and their incorporation into wider curriculum is essential. Thinking about these issues has benefited not only healthcare students in this university but is also informing the way we consider educational development more widely.

Professor Stuart Brand

Director of Learning and Teaching

Birmingham City University

ABOUT THE EDITORS

Matthew Aldridge, RN, RNT, M Ed, BSc (Hons), FHEA, is a senior lecturer in Acute Adult Nursing at the University of Wolverhampton. He has been instrumental in developing simulation as a learning and teaching methodology over the past seven years to enhance the delivery of healthcare education in a range of roles at Birmingham City University and, now in the School of Health and Wellbeing at the University of Wolverhampton. Matthew has worked regionally, nationally and internationally on the furtherance of the use simulation in healthcare education. He has a clinical background in emergency nursing and is passionate about the integration of high quality clinical skills education into the undergraduate healthcare curriculum.

Stephen Wanless, RN, RNT, BSc (Hons), PG Dip (Ed), is a senior academic and patient handling lead for the Faculty of Health at Birmingham City University. He has an interest in the integration of high end technology to support practical skills training and the development of e-learning.

Stephen has been leading the way in the development of management and patient handling simulation as learning and teaching tools to improve the delivery of transitional healthcare education at Birmingham City University. He has presented his work nationally and internationally in the use of management and patient handling simulation within healthcare education.

Stephen has a clinical background in critical care nursing and is passionate about the integration of high quality patient handling and management skills education into healthcare curricula.

NOTES ON THE CONTRIBUTORS

Amanda Andrews

RGN, BSc (Hons) CHN, DN PG Cert (Ed) MA (Ed)
Senior Lecturer, Faculty of Health, Birmingham City University

Tim Badger

RN, BSc (Hons), MSc
Senior Lecturer, Faculty of Health, Birmingham City University

Catherine Easthope

RGN, Respiratory Nurse Specialist, Walsall Healthcare NHS Trust

Alison Eddleston

RN (Adult), RNT, MBA, FHEA
Senior Lecturer in Acute, Operative and Critical Care Nursing, School of Health, University of Central Lancashire

Andrew Grindrod

RN (Adult), BSc (Hons) Nursing, BSc (Hons) Healthcare Practice
Specialist Practitioner Adult Nursing
Charge Nurse in Critical Care Outreach, University Hospitals Leicester (UHL)

Kim Harley

RGN, RNT, Cert Ed (FE), PG Cert, BSc Combined Studies, ONC, ENB 100
Senior Lecturer, Musculoskeletal Studies, Adult and Critical Care,
Birmingham City University

Meriel Hawker

RGN, MSc Pain Management, PG Dip (Ed)
Programme Director MSc Pain Management, School of Nursing and Midwifery,
Birmingham City University

Helen Holder

RN (Adult), DPSN, MSc Nutritional Support, MA (Ed)
Senior Lecturer Adult Nursing, Faculty of Health, Birmingham City University

Katie Holmes

BA (Hons) Theology, NVQ 4 Advice and Guidance
Careers Consultant (linked to Faculty of Health), Birmingham City University

Phil Jevon

RN, Bsc (Hons) PG Cert
Resuscitation and Clinical Skills Lead, Walsall Healthcare NHS Trust

Chris Jones

Dip HE Child Health Nursing, RN (Adult), BSc (Hons) Emergency Care
Senior Lecturer, Clinical Skills Child Health, Birmingham City University

Paul Knott

RN (Adult), BSc (Hons) Clinical Nursing Studies, PGCE
Resuscitation and Simulation Practitioner, Central Manchester University
Hospitals Foundation Trust

Lisa Lawton

MSc Training and Development RGN, Dip Nursing, BSc Nursing, PGCHE
Practice Placement Manager, Faculty of Education, Heart of England Foundation Trust

Robert Mapp

RN (Adult), BSc (Hons) Nursing Studies, PG Cert (Ed), PG Dip (Ed)
Senior Lecturer, Faculty of Health, Birmingham City University

Mandy Reynolds

EN, RGN, Diploma (Nursing Studies), PG Cert (Infection Prevention and Control)
Senior Infection Prevention and Control Nurse, Heart of England NHS Foundation Trust

Barry Ricketts

RN (Adult), BSc (Hons) Critical and Specialist Care-Cardiothoracic Nursing, PG
Cert (Ed), MSc Higher Professional Education
Senior Lecturer, Adult Nursing, School of Health and Social Care, Oxford Brookes
University

Bernie St Aubyn

BSc (Hons), RGN RM RHV DPS: N (CHS) MSc (PSM) PG Cert (Ed)
Senior Lecturer, Faculty of Health, Birmingham City University

Simon Steeves

Senior Lecturer, Mental Health Nursing, Birmingham City University

Paul Turner

RN (Adult), Dip Nursing (London), RNT, Cert (Ed), BSc, MSc
Senior Lecturer, Faculty of Health, Birmingham City University

Nathalie Turville

RGN, RSCN, DPNS, BSc (Hons), PG Cert (Ed), MSc
Senior Lecturer, Faculty of Health, Birmingham City University

Steve Wanless

BSc (Hons) Safety, Health and Environmental Management, Dip RG/RT, MCSP, SRP
Manual Handling Coordinator, Anonymous Foundation Trust, Manchester

Steven Webb

Clinical Skills and Simulation Technician, Walsall Healthcare NHS Trust

1

INTRODUCTION: BACKGROUND TO THE IMPORTANCE OF ESSENTIAL NURSING SKILLS

Stephen Wanless and Matthew Aldridge

The authors of this book have become renowned as experts in the teaching and development of clinical skills to healthcare students through simulation within the higher education arena. The team of academics and practitioners comprising the authorship of this book contribute to the development of simulation and practice-based teaching of many vocational qualifications, particularly in relation to pre-registration healthcare training courses.

This book has been written predominantly for academics and educators who work within the healthcare arena, in recognition of the challenges in the healthcare setting to deliver safe and competent care, and in order that the next generation of healthcare workers ease their transition to qualified practitioners; this book takes into account these issues and can serve as an essential resource for both healthcare academics and students. It is also a useful resource for educators who teach clinical skills and also for those who are involved in mentorship of students and those who are preceptors of newly qualified healthcare professionals.

The content of this book will provide the educator with the necessary skills to facilitate the progress of students with clinical and transitional skills. These skills are required by everyone studying healthcare and, with the context of healthcare evolving, every chapter has been linked with an example of a simulation.

The competency expected of healthcare professionals can vary from country to country as well as from one local healthcare institution to another. Some employers expect newly qualified staff to develop competency in some advanced skills within a short time of qualification. To ensure the reality shock caused during the transition from student to qualified practitioner is reduced the book has utilised simulation as a trigger to remind students of the practice that they have seen while in clinical practice.

The purpose of this book is to provide a resource that will truly meet the needs of the educator when teaching clinical and transitional skills through the use of simulation in content and style. It provides research-based evidence on how to perform and enhance skills and clinical procedures in a safe simulated context. It provides an optimal balance of theory and practice so that the reader will understand the rationale and evidence for the skill as well as how to teach it in a simulated environment.

The content is written in such a way as to aid learning and recall in the clinical environment through the use of simulation, helping the educator to assist the learner in gaining confidence and attaining competency. Educators often have to wade through large pieces of dense text; to guard against this here and to ensure a user-friendly layout, the text is full of many pedagogical features such as easy to find pictures, skills in table format, examples of simulation and a consistent approach to the formulation of each of the chapters.

The content of this book is divided into three sections with 21 chapters in total. We first look at the theory related to the use of simulation as a teaching tool. The text then covers the main aspects relating to the essential aspects of care that patients require, looking at common themes such as hygiene, drug administration and nutrition. The final part of the book covers the skills required to assist in the transition from student to qualified practitioner and looks at issues that may arise which the student may not have had exposure to, such as conflict management, incident reporting and breaking bad news. All skill-related chapters have an example of a simulation specific to that chosen skill for use or adaptation by the educator.

The book is meant as a useful and essential resource for anyone involved in healthcare education. The evidence base related to the skills that have been assembled for this edition, together with the unique range of contributors and their approaches, provides a rich source of information for a generation of healthcare professionals and their future practice.

2

DEFINING AND EXPLORING CLINICAL SKILLS AND SIMULATION-BASED EDUCATION

Matthew Aldridge

Studies have shown (Alinier et al., 2004; Lauder et al., 2008; Reilly and Spratt, 2007; Nursing and Midwifery Council (NMC), 2007) that the use of simulation in healthcare education curricula can have a positive impact upon learners' self-efficacy and self-confidence. Furthermore simulation allows learners to rehearse skills and enact scenarios that would be considered undesirable or unsafe to practise on real patients or clients for the first time (Broussard, 2008). Simulation can be a relatively resource-intensive learning and teaching methodology when compared with more traditional classroom-based didactic methods; however, there is an ever-increasing body of evidence which suggests simulation is not only valued by learners, but also is having a positive impact upon healthcare curricula and patient/client care enhancement.

FIDELITY OF SIMULATION

Fidelity is a widely discussed term when considering simulation and is described by Maran and Glavin (2003) in terms of engineering fidelity, in which the equipment reflects the true nature of the clinical setting, and psychological fidelity which refers to the authenticity the learner attributes to the setting, that is, their perceptions of its realism. Fidelity is an important consideration when designing and implementing simulation scenarios as it can impact upon the learning experience, both positively and negatively. Great care and effort could be placed in creating a technologically competent scenario using human patient simulators, however, if careful consideration has not been given to the fidelity of the actual scenario or expectations of the learners, then overall fidelity of the simulation may suffer.

NOMENCLATURE OF SIMULATION

The nomenclature and taxonomy of terms used within simulation are often debated, with some terms used interchangeably by different commentators. Very often the taxonomy of the fidelity of simulation is discussed in the terms of part-task training, low fidelity, medium fidelity and high fidelity simulation.

PART-TASK TRAINING

The term 'part-task devices' refers to equipment which allows the replication and rehearsal of a skill in isolation from the rest of an anatomical model. For example, intravenous therapy 'phantom arms' which allow venous cannulation and therapy, or 'phantom heads' which allow for dental training or the assessment of facial injuries.

These devices are useful as they are relatively cheap when compared with a full human patient simulator, have a reasonably good level of fidelity in replicating the real look and feel of the anatomical area in question, and provide skills rehearsal without risk to a real patient.

Roger Kneebone from Imperial College London has done some novel work on the use of 'hybrid models' which allow the adaptation of a part-task training device to be attached to a real person, thus allowing the rehearsal of both technical and non-technical skills simultaneously. This has been translated into a number of practice areas such as suturing, injection techniques, urinary catheterisation and female pelvic examination.

LOW FIDELITY SIMULATION

A low fidelity simulator may be just a static manikin or anatomical model, with no physiological signs or parameters, such as heart rate and blood pressure. However, this type of simulator may have some features such as an oral cavity or genitalia, which may allow the practice of some technical skills such as oral care or catheterisation. Another example may be the use of an orange to practise intramuscular injection techniques.

MEDIUM FIDELITY

Medium fidelity resources may include manikins which can replicate some physiological parameters or anatomical features. Examples of such devices are an electronic blood pressure training arm or a cannulation arm, which allow the learner to practise the skill with some degree of visual or tactile feedback.

HIGH FIDELITY SIMULATION

High fidelity resources include advanced physiological models and anatomical components which allow for the replication of medical and surgical conditions, often in the full context within which the situation would appear in the real-life setting. Examples may include advanced human patient simulators and advanced laparoscopic surgical trainers. Conversely, there may be no equipment used at all, and it may be the simulation of a communication scenario with a patient's/client's relative using a role player (Standardised Patient). Clearly the use of a human being to simulate a human interaction would give the highest degree of 'engineering fidelity', but the scenario and interaction would still require careful construction to ensure good 'psychological fidelity'.

TEACHING A CLINICAL SKILL

The teaching of clinical skills is sometimes – wrongly it must be stated – not given the same credence as other academic content in the curricula of undergraduate healthcare professionals. If we are to train competent, intelligent and enquiring healthcare professionals to fulfil a clinical role, then it is absolutely vital that they are equipped with both the academic and technical skills in order to carry out their role competently and confidently.

The system of 'master and apprentice' has often prevailed in the teaching of clinical skills in the past, though fortunately in recent years there has been a shift to recognise that learning will not necessarily happen just because a learner is exposed to a skill by a competent person in clinical practice, and indeed this is not considered a safe way to learn and rehearse the majority of clinical skills. A structured and curriculum-integrated approach should be taken to the teaching of clinical skills so that the theory and practice of a skill can be embedded in educational design and delivery.

Objective Structured Clinical Examinations (OSCEs) are now an established means of assessing a learner's ability to perform a clinical skill and are often included as a summative assessment somewhere in the majority of undergraduate healthcare curricula. OSCEs can be a reliable means of measuring a learner's understanding and performance of a clinical skill, though can be resource-intensive in the room, equipment and examiners required. Hence they need careful forethought and planning to run smoothly.

It is true that classroom-based didactic teaching requires a different skill set to that of the clinical skills laboratory setting, though this certainly should not infer any order of merit.

Peyton (1998) describes a widely used four-stage approach to teaching a skill:

1   Demonstration – Educator demonstrates the skill at normal speed without commentary
2   Deconstruction – The skill is broken down into its component parts while the educator gives commentary
3   Comprehension – The educator demonstrates the skill while the learner describes the steps
4   Performance – The learner demonstrates the skill while describing the steps.

The use of a detailed step-by-step lesson plan which explains each step in the skill and its rationale can be useful for both educator and learner to refer to, and will allow the learner to continue to rehearse or review the skill at a later time.

It is acknowledged (Hamilton, 2005; Oermann et al., 2010) that 'skills fade' or the degradation of retention of the ability to perform a clinical skill can occur as little as three months after the learning of a given skill. For this reason, repeated rehearsal and use of a skill would seem to be recommended in order to maintain competency. Repetition would appear to be vital in the teaching and learning of a skill as, in the educational setting, learners are frequently exposed to the teaching of a skill for as little as one hour, and then may not have the opportunity to revisit or rehearse that skill until they experience it on a 'real-life' patient in the clinical setting. Some educational delivery organisations have acknowledged the need to allow learners to practise clinical skills in their own time, in an area of low or remote supervision, thus allowing for repeated rehearsal and mastery of the psychomotor aspects of clinical skills.

There is a widespread belief that for skills- and simulation-based education to have its maximum impact it should be integrated into curricula, where possible, rather than being a stand-alone entity which may have limited value as a training event when delivered out of context to the curriculum as a whole.

PROBLEM-BASED LEARNING (PBL)

Problem-based learning offers the educator a means of providing simulation which requires very little resource. PBL is not appropriate for teaching technical skills; rather it allows the learner to exercise their cognitive, analytical and problem-solving skills by exploring a problem for themselves and determining appropriate solutions. Jones (2008: 213) lists one of the key benefits of PBL as: 'Increased motivation for the learner by focussing learning on real-life scenarios'.

Problem-based learning is often initiated by one or more 'trigger' sessions, which allow the educator to set the problem and feed-in information to learners about the complexity or nature of the problem, if necessary, at a later stage. Learners are then required to work alone or in groups to explore the problem and devise appropriate solutions. PBL can be used in both a formative and summative context, with learning objectives and assessment tasks set accordingly. As with other forms of simulation, the educator is required to act more as facilitator than teacher. Rather than imparting knowledge to the learner, the educator is required to manage the dynamics of the group, guide students in their reasoning and monitor the progress of learning. This type of facilitation deviates from the normal skill set of a didactic lecturer, and requires ground rules and training for the facilitator before expertise can be achieved.

PBL may also be combined with other modes of simulation, and some of the triggers used may be more hands-on simulations using role players (Standardised Patients) or human patient simulators.

THE USE OF ROLE-PLAY

Role-play can be described as a 'rehearsal for a future event', and when done in a controlled, structured and sensitive manner can be an immensely powerful learning tool. Role-play can be used to challenge and change attitudes of learners, involve a group in active learning, enhance critical thinking, and encourage synthesis and evaluation of information (Clark, 2008).

In the most basic form of role-play, it is possible to ask learners to take on the role of a particular patient or client and ask them to play this out with their colleagues. This may be suitable for short interactions, or to get learners to think outside of their own situations and ask them to consider how a patient or client would feel. However, downsides to this approach may be that learners feel uncomfortable with role-playing a particular role or do not have the prior experience to be able to put themselves in a given situation.

The use of professional role players, sometimes referred to as Standardised patients (SPs), is a concept that has been used in healthcare education, particularly in the undergraduate medical curriculum, for a number of years. SPs can be used in this setting to stage mock clinical assessments for history taking, clinical assessment and prescribing scenarios. They can also be used when sensitive situations need to be rehearsed, such as intimate examinations or the breaking of bad news. The use of SPs needs careful consideration and provision of appropriate training to function at this level, and in particular to give useful feedback to the learner. Suffice to say, a good actor does not necessarily make a good role player for healthcare education purposes.

It is essential that SPs are given some sort of preparation or training to fulfil their role, as they will often be required to re-tell comprehensive histories or symptoms which will convince the learner of a particular condition or situation. It is often desirable, and useful, for the SP to give feedback on the learner's performance following a scenario. For this reason, it is essential that SPs who are expected to give feedback are given some training on the use of feedback and debrief techniques. The feedback from a SP can be particularly rich and powerful as it gives the learner the perspective of a patient/client in a safe and low-risk environment.

EXPERT PATIENTS/CLIENTS/SERVICE USERS

The use of expert patients or service users can be helpful in relaying the perspective of the 'care receiver' to the 'care provider'. Personal experiences relayed by the service user of their experiences of healthcare can be rich and enlightening for the learner. However, careful consideration must be given to the psychological and emotional wellbeing of the service user. For instance, it would not be considered appropriate for a service user with mental health issues to play the role of a mental health service user in a simulation scenario, or a cancer patient to play the role of a person receiving the news about a diagnosis of cancer, due to the risk of distress this may cause to service users. The inclusion of service users as consultants in the design of curricula and the writing of simulation scenarios is becoming increasingly popular, as this can greatly increase the authenticity and fidelity of a scenario through the inclusion of first-hand experience. The inclusion of service users as stakeholders and consultants in education and care delivery should be welcomed, but requires careful management and organisation to ensure a coherent and safe approach to their involvement.

ELECTRONIC OR SCREEN-BASED SIMULATION

Electronic simulation programmes offer the advantage of the learner being able to learn away from the more formal setting of the clinical or skills laboratory. This method can allow for learning at the learner's own pace, with multiple attempts underpinned by the notion of self-directed learning. Depending upon the software platform and information technology (IT) infrastructure used, it could be possible for the student to access the resource through a web-based platform, allowing learners to use the resource wherever they have access to the Internet. One particular benefit of electronic simulations is that they can be done without the presence of an educator and can be used to free-up curriculum time by delivering educational content or preparing the student for practical face-to-face simulation. A downside of the use of screen-based simulation is the lack of fidelity and a disassociation a learner may feel between the simulation and the actual task; and this may be more the case with the generation that has grown up with video games and online resources that allow the user to be absorbed in an 'alternate reality'.

There is little evidence to suggest what is the best use of screen-based simulation, but it may be useful in the preparation of learners to exercise their cognitive abilities before practising the psychomotor domain in the skills lab or clinical practice setting.

HUMAN PATIENT SIMULATORS

A number of medium to high fidelity electronic human patient simulators exist and are available to educators, including: Laerdal Medical's 'SimMan'™ and 'SimBaby'™, METI's 'iSTAN'™ and Gaumard's 'HAL'™. These simulators are all designed to replicate the physiological observations, sounds, and in some cases, movements of a real human patient. The obvious advantage of this type of simulator is the high degree of fidelity offered to the user in their replication of a real patient, but without the risks of practising on live human patients. Such manikins can be programmed with pre-set scenarios which allow the facilitator to run a scenario with minimal set-up and intervention to the manikin's controls during the scenario. However, human patient simulators are also able to be used 'on the fly', whereby the facilitator can alter the manikin's vital signs and responses in real time, in response to the learner's actions or omissions as the scenario unfolds.

USE OF AUDIO VISUAL SYSTEMS

Various audio visual (AV) systems are available which will allow audio and video feeds to be recorded and/or broadcast simultaneously to another area. This can be particularly useful when large numbers of learners are involved, such as with undergraduate healthcare programmes, and can allow for large numbers of learners to participate in a scenario remotely. Such systems will also allow for 'event tagging' which allows the facilitator to highlight a particular incident during the recording of a scenario and then jump to that particular section later on during debrief while watching the video. The use of AV can be particularly useful to highlight behaviour or a performance which the learner was unaware of during the actual scenario.

If the use of AV systems is to be considered, it is highly advisable to involve an organisation's Information Technology (IT) department at the earliest opportunity so that they may assist with the consultation on the capabilities and limitations of an organisation's IT infrastructure before the purchase of any equipment. This will help to avoid issues of incompatibility of systems and equipment, and hopefully secure the buy-in of the IT department to maintain and support the equipment in the future. Ethical and legal consideration must also be given to the use, availability and storage of video images, in order to ensure that images are used appropriately and with the full consent of all parties involved.

GIVING FEEDBACK

It can certainly be argued that the debrief might be the most important part of any simulation exercise, as this is where the learner makes sense of what has happened during the simulation, and begins to explore and rationalise any learning that has taken place. Most importantly, the learner may have not yet noticed that a learning opportunity has taken place; therefore, it is essential that the facilitator is able to present such learning opportunities, with the assistance of AV playback perhaps, to the learner in a constructive and supportive manner.

DEBRIEF

Debrief should be:

- **Carried out as soon as practicable after the scenario ends** It is important to guide the debrief process to prevent candidates from deconstructing their own or their colleagues' performance without guidance
- **Structured** It is important that debrief has a structure to prevent it from becoming a rambling discussion or being hijacked by the agenda of a learner or their colleagues. A framework such as Kolb's (1984) experiential cycle of learning may be adapted to be used for simulated learning (see Figure 2.1)
- **Open and honest** Learners value an honest approach to debrief; 'sugar-coating' feedback or lying about a learner's performance in order to avoid hurting their feelings ultimately results in a poor learning experience. A less than honest debrief may also foster a false sense of security in a learner about their own performance
- **Constructive** It is important to be honest about a learner's feedback, but this must be done constructively and not become a character assassination of the learner. Inadequate and poor performance needs to be highlighted, but should be done in a manner which allows the candidate to frame this in a positive approach to improvement. Conversely, when a candidate displays good performance, this should be acknowledged and reflected upon so that lessons can be learnt for future practice.

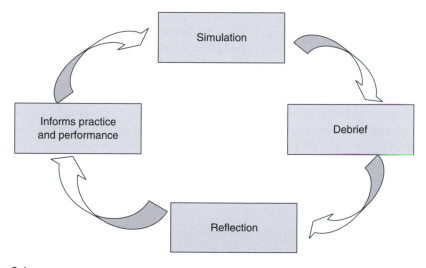

Figure 2.1

Adapted from Kolb's (1984) Cycle of Experiential Learning

- Debriefs must be diagnostic
- The organisation should create a supportive learning environment for debrief
- Team leaders and team members should be encouraged to be attentive of team work processes
- Team leaders should be educated on the art and science of leading team debriefs
- Ensure that team members feel comfortable during debriefs
- Focus on a few critical performance issues during the debrief process
- Describe specific teamwork interactions and processes that were involved in the team's performance
- Use objective indicators to support feedback
- Provide outcome feedback later and less frequently than process feedback
- Provide both individual and team-oriented feedback, but know when each is more appropriate
- Minimise the delay between task performance and feedback as much as possible
- Record conclusions made and goals set during the debrief to facilitate feedback in future debriefs

---

Figure 2.2

Salas et al., (2008) list a best evidence list of practices for successful debrief, reproduced here in Figure 2.2.

USING SIMULATION FOR ASSESSMENT

Simulation lends itself very well to formative assessment as it allows abundant opportunities to give detailed, directed and structured feedback on performance in a safe and supportive way. However, the use of simulation as a means of summative assessment is growing and, when used correctly and judiciously, can provide a reliable and robust means of assessment of learners' knowledge and performance.

An increasing interest is being shown in the use of simulation to accredit learners in 'high stakes' events, and has long been used in the testing and accreditation of professionals who are expected to perform Advanced Life Support (ALS) in the clinical environment. The growing use of simulation for competency assessment is developing in such areas as anaesthesia and surgery to accredit and revalidate the skills of healthcare professionals. While the assessment of skills involved in 'high-stakes' care delivery would appear to be desirable, it should not be forgotten that simulation has the potential to be a very powerful formative learning tool, and learners should be given every opportunity to rehearse skills in the simulation lab setting, accompanied by high-quality formative assessment and feedback, before exposure to summative assessment.

EDUCATOR/INSTRUCTOR PREPARATION

The creation and delivery of simulation sessions can at first appear a daunting undertaking to educators who have not used this method before. However, this need not be the case and careful preparation is often the key to allaying fears. If the expectation is for other educators to run a scenario they have not created then, at the very least, an instruction manual should be provided. This manual should provide:

- Learning aims and objectives
- Equipment and resources list
- A background to the simulation and context (scene-setter)
- A description of roles and cues to be used by Standardised Patients (if used)
- Prompts for learners and how to involve them in the simulation
- A description of settings for electronic manikins and human patient simulators, with instructions how to programme (if used)
- A step-by-step guide to how each scenario or step of the simulation unfolds
- A guide to debriefing the simulation, with key learning and discussion points
- A resource pack with any additional material, for example, relevant guidelines or notes and charts to be used.

McGaghie et al. (2010: 53) make the observation that 'Clinical experience is not a proxy for simulation instructor effectiveness.' This acknowledges that even the most accomplished and experienced clinicians, who intend to embark upon simulation-based educational delivery, require some sort of preparation in order for them to become effective teachers or instructors, and in order to capitalise upon their skills and experience in the classroom or skills and simulation lab. There appears to be a gap in the validation and accreditation of simulation instructors and facilitators. It has long been acknowledged in education that a Post Graduate Certificate in Education (PG Cert Ed) is an accepted and respected qualification to prepare some-one to teach in further and higher education, but no uniform comparable qualifica-tion exists in the preparation of simulation instructors/facilitators. There is a growing interest in the use of simulation for the accreditation and validation/revali-dation of healthcare professionals and, if this is to be the case, there is then a strong argument for the creation of uniform programmes of preparation to ensure validity and reliability in this form of assessment and accreditation.

Familiarisation training, particularly when using electronic equipment and human patient simulators, is a valuable means of helping to allay fears and maximise the use of equipment. Facilitators may not feel comfortable using a particular piece of equipment simply because they are not familiar with its controls or functions.

Conversely, neophyte educators and instructors may also benefit from instruction in the pedagogical models of simulation, including: Lave and Wenger's (1990) situated cognition, Benner's (1984) 'novice to expert' model and Tanner's (2006) theory of clinical judgement. Reflective insights such as Kolb's model and Schon's (1983) 'Reflective Practitioner' have also been combined with pedagogical frameworks to create models for simulation.

It may be helpful to consider the component parts of healthcare education delivery as a cyclical model when designing simulation.

LEARNING OUTCOMES

Design of all learning and teaching experiences should begin with setting learning outcomes and using these as a 'peg' or framework upon which to 'hang' the rest of the content.

Assessment

The learning activities should be closely aligned with both the learning outcomes and the assessment methods (Biggs, 1999) to ensure that the learning has meaning, value and purpose.

Simulation activities

This may include part-task training, low and medium to high fidelity simulation opportunities.

Feedback

The inclusion of high-quality feedback in the form of: debriefs, informal feedback or more formal feedback, such as written feedback following an OSCE.

Opportunity for Skills Rehearsal

There should be an opportunity for learners to rehearse skills in their own time, with low or remote supervision, if deemed necessary, in order to combat skills fade and reinforce deeper learning.

Other Learning Activities

This may include Problem-based Learning (PBL), didactic delivery or screen-based electronic learning and can be used to deliver theoretical components, or support cognitive development.

Skills of the Educator/Facilitator

Do the educators or facilitators involved in the delivery and support of learning have the appropriate skills needed or is development required. How will you ensure parity, and validity and reliability of learning and teaching delivery among educators, i.e. core lesson plans or instructor manuals?

EVALUATING THE IMPACT OF SIMULATION

A commonly utilised framework for the evaluation of educational delivery upon pre-set outcomes is Kirkpatrick's (1979) Hierarchy of Evaluation (see Figure 2.4).

Kirkpatrick's model details the levels of evaluation from the reaction of the learner through to impact upon the learner's behaviour and its impact upon systems or processes.

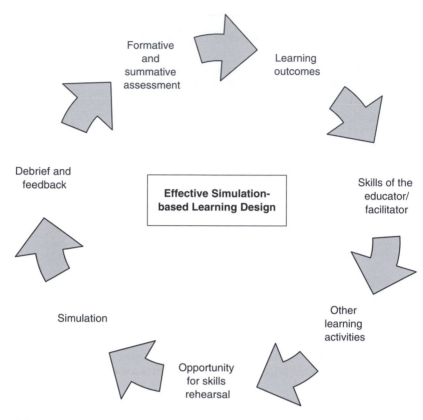

Figure 2.3

It is acknowledged that considerable difficulty exists in the measurement of outcomes of simulation-based educational delivery. It is relatively easy to measure a learner's self-efficacy pre- and post-simulation (Kirkpatrick levels one and two); however, it is more difficult to reliably measure the impact of simulation-based educational delivery on patient/client outcomes in the clinical area (Kirkpatrick levels three and four), often due to the multi-factorial nature of the clinical environment and patient/client situation. It could be said that it is difficult to measure the impact of any educational delivery upon patient/client outcome, though the stakes may be much higher for simulation as often significant resources and financial support are required to initiate and sustain simulation-based delivery, and some education and care providers may decide that sufficient evidence to support the cost–benefit ratio exists. Some authors (Phillips, 1996) have argued for the inclusion of a 'fifth level' to the Kirkpatrick model of evaluation, a 'Return on Investment' level, where the benefit to the organisation or outcome is measured in terms of the level of benefit it provides in relation to the resources invested. This may become increasingly important as the fiscal climate in healthcare and education demands a clearer cost–benefit ratio on an ever-decreasing availability of funding.

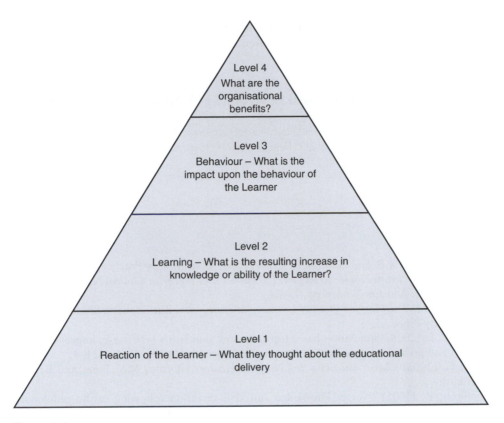

Figure 2.4

Source: Kirkpatrick (1979) Hierarchy of Evaluation

Clearly a more sustained and sophisticated effort is needed with the evaluation of simulation-based educational delivery to determine the best and most cost-effective ways of delivering benefit, both to the learners and to patients/clients.

CONCLUSION

Simulation can be an immensely powerful learning and teaching tool, but is in no way a 'magic bullet', which when fired in the direction of a course or curriculum, will instantly solve all issues. Simulation, like all other learning and teaching methodologies, must be used cautiously and judiciously when designing a learning experience. Consideration must be given to the learning styles and levels of the intended learners and the resources, time and expertise available to the educator.

This book may be particularly useful to both learner and educator, as it not only demonstrates a raft of clinical skills, procedures and a broad knowledge base, but also highlights how the learning and teaching methodologies involved in simulation can be used to enhance the learner experience.

USEFUL ORGANISATIONS AND NETWORKS FOR FURTHER INFORMATION

Association for Simulated Practice in Healthcare (ASpiH): http://www.aspih.org.uk/
Society in Europe for Simulation Applied to Medicine (SESAM): http://www.sesam-web.org/
Society for Simulation in Healthcare (SSiH): http://www.ssih.org

---

REFERENCES

Alinier, G., Hunt, W.B. and Gordon, R. (2004) *Nurse Education in Practice*, 4 (3): 200–7.

Benner, P. (1984) *From Novice to Expert: Excellence and Power in Clinical Nursing Practice.* Menlo Park: Addison-Wesley. pp. 13–34.

Biggs, J. (1999) *Teaching for Quality Learning at University.* Buckingham: SRHE and Open University Press.

Broussard, L. (2008) 'Simulation-based learning: how simulators help nurses improve clinical skills and preserve patient safety', *Nursing for Women's Health*, 12 (6): 521–4.

Clark, C. (2008) *Classroom Skills for Nurse Educators.* Boston, MA: Jones and Bartlett Publishers.

Hamilton, R. (2005) 'Nurses knowledge and skill retention following cardio pulmonary resuscitation training: a review of the literature', *Journal of Advanced Nursing*, 51 (3): 288–97.

Jones, W. (2008) 'Problem-based learning for simulation in healthcare', in R. Riley (ed.), *Manual of Simulation in Healthcare.* Oxford: Oxford University Press, pp. 213–226.

Kirkpatrick, D.L. (1979) 'Techniques for evaluating training programs', *Training and Development Journal*, 33 (6): 78–92.

Kolb, D.A. (1984) *Experiential Learning Experience as a Source of Learning and Development.* NJ: Prentice Hall.

Lauder, W., Holland, K., Roxburgh, M., Topping, K., Watson, R., Johnson, M. and Porter, M. (2008) 'Measuring competence, self-reported competence and self-efficacy in pre-registration students', *Nursing Standard*, 22 (20): 35–43.

Lave, J. and Wenger, E. (1990) *Situated Learning: Legitimate Peripheral Participation.* Cambridge: Cambridge University Press.

Maran, N.J. and Glavin, R.J. (2003) 'Background low- to high-fidelity simulation: a continuum of medical education', *Medical Education*, 37 (1): 22–8.

McGaghie, W., Issenberg, B., Petrusa, E. and Scalese, R. (2010) 'A critical review of simulation-based medical education research: 2003–2009', *Medical Education*, 44: 50–63.

Nursing and Midwifery Council (2007) Simulation and Practice Learning Project. Outcome of a Pilot Study to Test the Principles for Auditing Simulated Practice Learning Environments in the Pre-registration Nursing Programme.

Oermann, M., Kardong-Edgren, S., McColgan, J., Hurd, D., Haus, C., Snelson, C., Hallmark, B.F., Rogers, N., Kuerschner, D., Ha, Y., Tennant, M., Dowdy, S. and Lamar, J. (2010) 'Advantages and barriers to use of HeartCode BLS with voice advisory manikins for teaching nursing students', *International Journal of Nurse Education Scholarship*, 7 (1): Article 26.

Peyton, J. (1998) *Teaching and Learning in Medical Practice*. Rickmansworth: Manticore Europe Ltd.

Phillips, J. (1996) 'How much is the training worth?', *Training and Development*, 50 (4): 20–4.

Reilly, A. and Spratt, C. (2007) 'The perceptions of undergraduate student nurses of high-fidelity simulation-based learning: a case report from the University of Tasmania', *Nurse Education Today*, 27: 542–50.

Salas, E., Klein, C., King, H., Salisbury, M., Augenstein, J.S., Birnbach, D.J., Robinson, D.W. and Upshaw, C. (2008) 'Debriefing medical teams: 12 evidence-based best practices and tips', *Joint Commission Journal on Quality and Patient Safety*, 34: 518–27.

Schon, D. (1983) *The Reflective Practitioner: How Professionals Think in Action*. London: Temple Smith.

Tanner, C. (2006) 'The next transformation: clinical education', *Journal of Nursing Education*, 45: 99–100.

3

PATIENT ASSESSMENT: THE ABCDE APPROACH TO PATIENT ASSESSMENT AND EARLY WARNING SCORING SYSTEMS

Andrew Grindrod

Aim

The aim of this chapter is to give an overview of the ABCDE approach to prioritisation of patient care.

Objectives

The healthcare professional will:

- Understand the term 'track and trigger scoring system'.
- Be able to calculate an Early Warning Score (EWS) based on local EWS chart.
- Be able to discuss the ABCDE approach to patient assessment and each of its individual components.

INTRODUCTION TO PATIENT ASSESSMENT USING THE ABCDE APPROACH

EARLY WARNING SCORING (EWS) SYSTEMS

Within hospital at any given time there are large numbers of patients with widely varying levels of dependence. These may range from the patient who is physically well awaiting a care package to the acutely unwell individual requiring complex intervention. To complicate matters further this variety may be seen within the same ward, or even in the same bay, being cared for by the same healthcare professionals.

Recognising the acutely ill patient or those at risk of deterioration can be problematic. This is supported by the National Confidential Enquiry into Patient Outcome and Death (NCEPOD) report 'An acute problem' in 2005 (Simpson, 2005). They found a number of issues surrounding the care of acutely ill patients including: suboptimal care due to failure of organisation, lack of knowledge, failure to appreciate clinical urgency, lack of supervision, and failure to seek advice. Furthermore, they found that in the patients admitted to an Intensive Care Unit, those who had received suboptimal care prior to admission had an increased mortality rate which was approximately double that of those in the well-managed group (Simpson, 2005). When NCEPOD examined the cases of 'unexpected' in-hospital cardiac arrests they found that, 'many patients had clearly recorded evidence of marked physiological deterioration prior to the event without any appropriate action being taken in many cases' (Simpson, 2005). These points emphasise the need for a robust method of identifying patients at risk of deterioration linked to a framework for escalation in care, frequency of observation and referral pathway ensuring the appropriate care of the patient by professionals with the relevant skills.

Early Warning Scoring systems (EWS) are a form of track and trigger system and were designed in an attempt to identify patients at risk of deterioration, prompting early identification treatment and appropriate referral of the acutely ill patient. The observations are charted and a score is generated, which then triggers a particular response.

The level of response very much depends on the score and may range from an increase in the frequency of observations to requesting a review from the patient's medical/surgical team or a Critical Care Outreach Team. This helps to ensure that members of the healthcare team refer patients in a timely and appropriate fashion in response to a trigger score, in order to facilitate prompt intervention and maximise the potential for patient improvement. Often the system used is a multiple parameter system.

The minimum patient physiological parameters to be recorded that were suggested by NICE (2007) include respiratory rate, systolic blood pressure, temperature, heart rate, level of consciousness and oxygen saturation. There should be consideration to increasing this to include hourly urine output, biochemical analysis and pain assessment in some circumstances.

Some track and trigger charts do not score a patient on their oxygen saturations but make reference to a range of oxygen saturations for the healthcare provider to aim for. Typically the patient scores a 0–3 on each physiological parameter. Therefore, if five physiological parameters are scored the minimum a patient would score would be 0 and the maximum would be 15. In the example included in the text the temperature scores a maximum of 2, making the total score 14. Action may depend on total score, as the scores for each parameter are added together, or on a high score in one particular parameter. It may be more concerning for a patient to score a 3 in respiratory rate alone (respiratory rate would be greater than 30 per minute), than a total of 3 – one in each of respiratory rate, heart rate and temperature.

Track and trigger systems have existed in a variety of forms for a number of years, and in recent years have been advocated by the National Institute for Health and Clinical Excellence (NICE). In 2007 they published their guidance on acutely ill patients in hospital (NICE clinical guideline 50). NICE suggested that 'physiological track and trigger systems should be used to monitor all adult patients in acute hospital settings'. Further to this the score denotes the response, i.e. the greater the score the higher the level of response. It was recommended that classifying the patient into low, medium and high score groups would be beneficial, and suggested the actions and referrals for each group (NICE, 2007).

ABCDE APPROACH TO PATIENT ASSESSMENT

The ABCDE approach has been fostered by a number of emergency intervention courses such as the Advanced Life Threatening Event Recognition and Treatment (ALERT™), Advanced Life Support (ALS), Care of the Critically Ill Medical Patient (CRIMP) and Care of the Critically Ill Surgical Patient (CRISP). The basic premise is not to move on from A to B and so on until identified problems have been addressed or resolved. This approach should be used in all patients who have been identified as acutely unwell or at risk of deterioration, irrespective of whether an EWS system is used in the patient's location. The sequence from A to E is deliberate in that an obstructed airway will lead to the death of a patient more quickly than a fast respiratory rate, for example.

The benefits of such a systematic approach include:

- Maximum retention of information on the part of the healthcare professional
- More thorough patient assessment, ensuring aspects do not get missed
- Avoidance of fragmented approach that may lead to further deterioration
- A framework to go into any given situation with and treat the patient appropriately
- Increased appreciation of how acutely unwell a patient is and the appropriateness for referral to other specialities
- Prompt intervention while awaiting other specialist advice/review thereby limiting wasted time in treating the patient, which can be critical.

When assessing the patient using the ABCDE system the health professional should utilise a look, listen and feel approach.

(Continued)

PATIENT OBSERVATION CHART / MEDICAL EARLY WARNING SYSTEM — NHS

University Hospitals of Leicester
NHS Trust

Please complete or affix label

Name:	ADMITTING WARD:
Hospital No:	Date:
Date of Birth:	Moved to: Date:
Consultant:	Moved to: Date:
NHS No:	Moved to: Date:

Allergies:

Urinalysis	pH:	Protein:	Blood:	Leucocytes:	Glucose:	Ketones:	Nitrates:

BM Admission

If >8 or <3, inform nurse in charge

Score	3	2	1	0	1	2	3
Heart Rate	<40	-	40-50	51 - 100	101 - 110	111 - 129	≥130 or >130
Resp Rate	<8	-	-	8 - 20	21 - 25	26 - 30	>30
Temp C		≤35 or <35	35.1 - 36	36.1 - 37.9	38 - 38.4	≥38.5 or >38.5	
CNS	New weakness	Confused or agitated		Alert	Responds to voice	Responds to pain	Unresponsive
Systolic BP	<80	80 - 89	90 - 109	110 - 160	161 - 180	181 - 200	>200

N.B. IF ANY PATIENT SCORES GREATER THAN 0, A TRAINED NURSE MUST BE INFORMED

Score 1 - 2
* Inform a Trained Nurse, who must assess the patient
* Trained nurse to decide if patient requires BD or 4 hourly observations
* Patient requires a minimum of BD observations
* Establish target saturations and administer oxygen accordingly
* In ED: Inform co-ordinator. If < 90 consider ER space

Score = 3
* Trained Nurse to re-check observations
* Increase frequency of patient observations to at least 2 hourly
* Establish target saturations and administer oxygen accordingly
* In ED: Observations must be recorded hourly. Discuss with patient co-ordinator

Score is 3 in ONE parameter
* Trained Nurse to re-check observations
* Increase frequency of patient observations to at least 1 hourly
* Commence strict fluid balance monitoring and consider catheterisation
* Nurse to contact FY1/FY2 and inform them that patient requires medical review ASAP
* Establish target saturations and administer oxygen accordingly
* In ED: Senior review. Does the patient need ER space?

Total Score is 4 or above
* Trained Nurse to re-check observations
* Increase frequency of patient observations to at least 1 hourly
* Commence strict fluid balance monitoring and consider catheterisation
* Nurse to contact FY1/FY2 and inform them that patient requires urgent medical review
* FY1/FY2 should seek senior advice as needed from parent team Registrar and/or Consultant
* Establish target saturations and administer oxygen accordingly
* In ED: Senior review and prioritise patient. Observations ½ hourly

Total Score is greater than 4
* Trained Nurse to re-check observations
* Hourly observations
* Immediate review by senior doctor (own team or on-call out-of-hours)
* Registrar may need to discuss patient with own Consultant if necessary
* Consider contacting Critical Care Outreach Team or on-call ITU Team, if appropriate.
* Establish target saturations and administer oxygen accordingly
* In ED: Observations ¼ hourly. Patient needs ER bed

* If at any time there is no response from the medical team or the patient's condition is still causing concern, the next most senior doctor should be contacted.
* If at any time the patient is at risk of cardio-respiratory arrest activate the resuscitation team by dialling 2222.
* If a patient is known/suspected to be pregnant, inform Labour Ward Co-ordinator for obstetric/midwife assessment.
Ext 6541/2-LRI Ext 4805-LGH

Summary of interventions

Name: _____ Hosp. No: _____ Ward: _____ Site: _____

Date:	Time:		Total EWS:	
Summary:
Signature: _____ Print Name: _____

| Date: | Time: | | Total EWS: | |
Summary:
Signature: _____ Print Name: _____

| Date: | Time: | | Total EWS: | |
Summary:
Signature: _____ Print Name: _____

| Date: | Time: | | Total EWS: | |
Summary:
Signature: _____ Print Name: _____

| Date: | Time: | | Total EWS: | |
Summary:
Signature: _____ Print Name: _____

| Date: | Time: | | Total EWS: | |
Summary:
Signature: _____ Print Name: _____

| Date: | Time: | | Total EWS: | |
Summary:
Signature: _____ Print Name: _____

| Date: | Time: | | Total EWS: | |
Summary:
Signature: _____ Print Name: _____

| Date: | Time: | | Total EWS: | |
Summary:
Signature: _____ Print Name: _____

| Date: | Time: | | Total EWS: | |
Summary:
Signature: _____ Print Name: _____

(Continued)

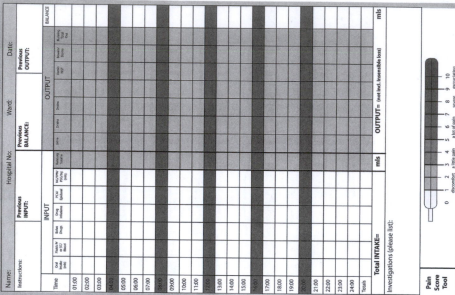

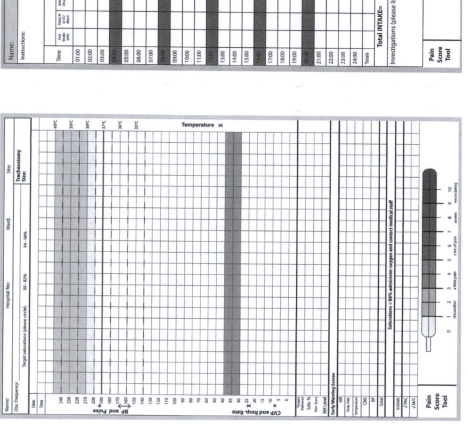

Figure 3.1

Source: University Hospitals of Leicester, Surgical Early Warning System, designed by C. Barclay, Critical Care Outreach Lead. Reproduced with permission of UHL and C. Barclay Critical Care Outreach Lead.

AIRWAY

Management of the airway is an essential skill to have within the resuscitation or medical emergency team. 'Prompt assessment, with control of the airway and provision of ventilation is essential' (Nolan et al., 2008: 41). Lack of oxygen leads to anaerobic respiration at a cellular level, this in turn produces an acidosis as lactate is produced. Life threatening hypoxia, if not addressed promptly and effectively, can result in a hypoxic brain injury. Healthcare professionals may be presented with airway emergencies at any time in their career, from student to experienced practitioner, and it is essential that individuals are able to deal with these emergencies in a timely and effective manner.

In order to resolve an airway issue there are a number of airway adjuncts at our disposal. Initial action should always be to provide a patent airway and 100% oxygen as soon as possible after an airway issue is identified. Assessment of a patient airway may be as easy as speaking to the patient and gaining a verbal response. However, the ability to use airway adjuncts in an emergency situation is a necessary skill for healthcare professionals caring for acutely unwell patients. The insertion of oropharyngeal and nasopharyngeal airways (see Figure 3.2) is an essential skill taught on many courses focussed on caring for the acutely ill patient or on resuscitation. Alternative actions are the use of a head tilt chin lift, or a jaw thrust.

BREATHING

The natural progression from airway is to breathing. Although this is one of the most accurate indicators of deterioration, it is often poorly monitored and recorded. According to Cretikos et al. (2008: 658), 'A raised respiratory rate is a strong and

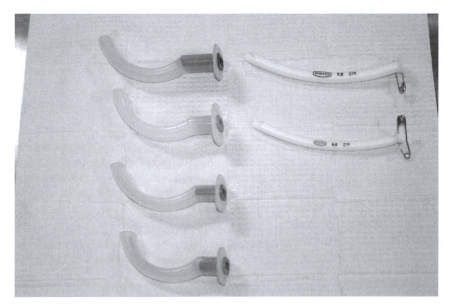

Figure 3.2

Table 3.1

Action	Rationale
Assess respiratory rate (covertly) – one breath in and one out = one respiration Assess respirations over full minute	• Early detection of deterioration
Do not talk to the patient or make them aware you are checking this	• Patient awareness may lead them to change the way they are breathing
Look at the patient	• Indicators of discomfort such as pursed lips breathing • Severe musculoskeletal abnormalities such as kyphosis or scoliosis will significantly impact patient's ability to generate good volumes

Check trachea centrally located	• Deviation may indicate:
	  o Tension pneumothorax
	  o Lung lobe collapse

Assess adequate depth of respiration – Introduce self and explain procedure to patient Expose the patient's chest, place hands at either side of chest to feel expansion	• Put patient more at ease, gain consent • External signs of disease? • Nil movement = airway obstruction, intervene and call emergency assistance • Assess the patient's ability to generate adequate tidal volumes for gas exchange. Reduced volume may indicate collapse, consolidation, large pleural effusion or poor inspiratory effort
Look for use of accessory muscles and intercostal recession	• Indicator of increased respiratory effort and patient deterioration
Look and feel for equal expansion	• Unequal – flail segment, plugging off of airway, consolidation, collapse
Feel for tactile fremitus (vibrations under hand when placed on patient's chest)	• Demonstrates secretions present
Look at pattern of breathing	• Abnormal breathing patterns, such as Cheyne-stokes; Kussmaul's respirations – indicate severe acidosis that requires addressing immediately
Listen to the patient: Able to complete full sentences Gurgles	• Inability to do this indicates respiratory distress • Secretions present in upper airway – may require suction to remove • Indicates narrowing of the airways which may require intervention – nebulizers or inhalers. May be cardiac in origin

(Continued)

Table 3.1   (Continued)

Action	Rationale
Wheeze	• Indicates partial airway obstruction requiring immediate intervention
Snoring	• Using stethoscope, listen to the apices, mid-zones and bases both anterior and posterior
Auscultate chest	• More subtle information such as wheezes, pleural rubs, bronchial breathing over consolidation
Ask patient if they are coughing and expectorating any secretions and the nature of them	• Patient may give evidence of chest infection, if thick secretions – needs physiotherapy, humidification +/– saline nebulisation

specific predictor of serious adverse events such as cardiac arrest and unplanned intensive care unit admission'. When assessing a patient's respiratory rate health professionals should be strongly encouraged to count this over a full minute without talking. The accepted normal respiratory rate is 14–18 breaths/minute (Mallett and Dougherty, 2001: 418). There are a wide variety of health issues both acute and chronic that can affect respiratory rate so a baseline is always useful. In many cases the patient will score higher for respiratory rate on their EWS, but if they would score higher normally when healthy this should be taken into account and goals set accordingly. If something appears wrong, further investigation usually reveals a clinical reason for this. The look, listen and feel approach to assessment continues throughout all the categories, so the health professional should adhere to this when assessing a patient's respiratory system.

CIRCULATION

Proceeding from breathing we come to circulation. This covers the aspects as listed in Table 3.2.

DISABILITY

A variety of aspects should be examined when working through the disability component of the A to E assessment. A scoring tool of some description should be utilised such as the Glasgow Coma Scale. The author, however, would advocate the use of the AVPU assessment tool where the patient's level of response is gauged – Alert, V responds to voice, P responds to painful stimuli or Unresponsive. There is a very strong link between level of consciousness and the airway. A problem with one may rapidly affect the other.

Table 3.2

Procedure	Rationale
Heart rate – feel radial pulse for one minute although in a collapsed patient a central pulse such as the carotid pulse should be palpated (see Figure 3.3)	• Detect rate – over one whole minute, assess character, regular, irregular, bounding, thready • If tachycardic, bradycardic +/– irregular consider 12 lead ECG • Tachycardia – consider hypovolaemia, shock, sepsis, primary cardiac cause • Bradycardia – consider heart block, overdose, if young and very fit, may be normal • Bounding – consider sepsis • Slow rising – consider aortic stenosis
Blood pressure	• If using automated method, and in any doubt of accuracy of reading or pulse is irregular check manually using sphygmomanometer. Consider what is normal for the patient and contrast with current blood pressure, aim should be to maintain the norm for the patient • Low – consider all forms of shock, end organ perfusion may be compromised leading to organ dysfunction e.g. renal failure. Fluid resuscitation may be indicated • High – is the patient in pain or distress? Not had usual antihypertensive or not absorbing them • Note – low blood pressure is a late indication of deterioration therefore speed is of the essence
Temperature – use tempadot or tympanic thermometer	• Hypothermia – consider environment, shut down secondary to shock and blood loss. May use warming methods such as warming blankets or warmed fluids – caution, increasing temperature too quickly can lead to vasodilatation and hypotension in an already compromised patient • Hyperthermia – consider infective process, take into account environmental temperature, number of blankets, warming systems that may be in place
Capillary refill time (CRT): Peripheral – press on finger nail for five seconds. Central – press on skin of sternum for five seconds. Should return to pink within two seconds	• Prolonged (CRT) indicates poor perfusion, may be secondary to low blood pressure, low circulating volume or poor perfusion for other reasons, e.g. peripheral vascular disease, Raynaud's disease • If skin appears mottled they may be peripherally shut down indicating that blood supply is being diverted to vital organs

(Continued)

Table 3.2 (Continued)

Procedure	Rationale
Urine Output >0.5mls/kg/hr (ALERT course handbook, Smith, 2003b)	• If not passed urine in 6–12 hours assess urine output which may require urinary catheterisation • If acutely unwell – hourly urine measurements and documentation • The kidneys 'auto regulate', to the patient's usual blood pressure range and hence a patient with hypertension may require a significantly higher mean arterial pressure than someone without it in order for the kidneys to filter adequately. Low urine output – consider increasing fluid intake. If absent rule out blockage in the system, e.g. obstructed catheter, consider ultrasound renal tract for stones, hydronephrosis
IV access	• If acutely unwell/deteriorating – ensure adequate functioning IV access. Assess for signs of infection
Fluid administration	• Appropriate fluids and volume replacement. May need to make reference to blood tests such as urea and electrolytes • Question the patient about if they are drinking and if so an estimate as to how much, check the mucous membranes to see if they are moist or dry – each giving an indication as to the patient's hydration state. There may be other indications as to the patient's fluid balance such as oedema that may not be noted until the assessment progresses to exposure • Accurate fluid balance is invaluable in assessing a patient's hydration state
Antibiotics	• Is the patient on any antimicrobial therapy? Is it an appropriate antimicrobial for the identified/presumed infection? Is it the correct dose? Has the patient received it? In severe sepsis we know that for every hour's delay in administration of antibiotics over the next six hours there is an associated increase in mortality of 7.6%/hour (Kumar et al., 2006). This is on top of a mortality of 30% – 50% already linked to severe sepsis • Caution – not all patients with sepsis become pyrexial
Pallor	• Is the patient pale? This may have implications for the patient's haemoglobin level and hence their blood pressure and oxygen-carrying capacity
Blood tests	• Check recent results to gather further evidence as to the patient's condition, e.g. low haemoglobin possibly indicating blood loss, or raised urea and creatinine which may indicate acute kidney injury

- A   Alert – patient is awake and alert
- V   Voice – responds to voice
- P   Pain – responds to painful stimulus. If patient does not respond to voice at a loud level, use painful stimulus. Airway support may be required
- U   Unresponsive – does not respond to anything. Airway support may be required

Hypoglycaemia is a common cause of decreased level of consciousness that is relatively easily remedied, but often overlooked in an emergency situation. In any patient with a decreased level of consciousness it is quick and easy to take a blood sugar measurement. Should the patient be hypoglycaemic then a glucose replacement substance should be used in line with local policies; these may include an oral preparation if able to take orally or, if not, the administration of 50% glucose via a large bore cannula in a large vein may be necessary. This may rapidly reverse the hypoglycaemia and, with it, an airway issue that may coexist.

If necessary, in the acute hypoglycaemic episode airway support must also be given. Not all reasons for decreased conscious level are so easily addressed, therefore the healthcare professional should also consider other reasons that may warrant further investigation. The pupils should be examined for diameter, equality in size and reactivity to light. Unequal and/or lack of reactivity to light can indicate an intra-cerebral event and should prompt the need for a CT scan, while pinpoint pupils may require further investigation into medications that may have been taken – both prescribed and non-prescribed – particularly those of an opiate derivation. If this is thought to be the case, then a reversal agent such as naloxone may be required, and it should be remembered that naloxone 'has short duration of action – repeated doses or infusion may be necessary to reverse the effects of opioids with longer duration of action' (British National Formulary, 2009: 702). When considering the transfer of a patient with a potential neurological injury it is vital to consider the potential for deterioration and arrange for staff with appropriate skills to attend. As there is such a close link between conscious level and the airway, members of staff with airway skills should be included, often the anaesthetist.

EXPOSURE

Exposure of the patient to conclude the A to E assessment should be done with an emphasis on maintaining the patient's dignity. There is also the potential with prolonged exposure for the patient to become hypothermic and every effort should be made to avoid this. As with the other areas of the A to E assessment, examination is by using a look, listen and feel approach (see Table 3.3). Essentially, when in the category of exposure the health professional should examine 'everything else'.

A basic knowledge of how the abdominal areas are described will be required when noting your findings. Anything that appears abnormal or any pain should be noted and used, with the other evidence gathered throughout the assessment, in order to identify current issues/problems. As the A to E assessment draws to a close there should be little or nil emergency interventions remaining as these should have been addressed as they were identified working through this systematic approach.

Table 3.3

Procedure	Rationale
Look	• Look for any abnormalities such as scars, deformities, rashes, lumps, open wounds, and discolouration such as the white, waxy appearance of an under perfused limb or any obvious hernias • A mottled appearance can indicate that the patient is extremely shut down; this is a reflection of critical illness, time is of the essence in this situation • Bed linen should be removed/moved to rule out any hidden blood loss such as per rectum or per vagina
Listen	• Listen to the abdomen for evidence of bowel sounds, the sounds heard or lack thereof may give support to the potential diagnosis. 'Early mechanical bowel obstruction produces hyperactive peristaltic waves proximal to the mechanical obstruction. These waves are increased in frequency and force and produce a concomitant increase in bowel sounds with characteristic "rushes". As the bowel gradually dilates with gas and fluid, the bowel sounds become high pitched and tinkling, and there may be periods of hypoactive bowel sounds that alternate with hyperperistaltic rushes. These rushes correlate with the increased peristaltic activity. Finally, in late intestinal obstruction there may be loss of all bowel sounds due to loss of peristaltic activity from vascular compromise.' (Walker et al., 1990)
Feel	• Palpate the abdomen – ask the patient if there are any areas that are particularly tender before commencing. Palpation should be done in a systematic way. Start in one area and work around the entirety of the abdomen palpating lightly initially and then repeat pressing deeper using a rolling motion and placing one hand over the other to provide the pressure • The practitioner should not dig in, prod and probe with the fingertips, rather progressively increase pressure using the flat of the hand. This will elicit any pain that may be present; however, stoical individuals may try to conceal their pain so the healthcare practitioner should watch the patient's face for evidence of any discomfort during the examination. The site of any pain should be noted and scored using local pain scoring systems • Feel any abnormalities to ascertain the size, shape, mobility • Is any pain elicited? • Feel other areas also that may reveal abnormal findings that were not evident on looking • This is just as relevant when examining joints, where range of movement should be observed, noting any movement which causes pain • Feel for any crepitation at the joints or areas of swelling and heat • Remember the five Fs when examining an abdomen – fat, fluid, flatus, faeces and foetus • Explore for any organ abnormality such as that of an enlarged liver or spleen • Feel for the urinary bladder, if a patient has not passed urine and a bladder is felt then there is an obstruction to urine flow that needs to be resolved

However, a great deal more can be learnt from the patient's notes and history that may be useful in gathering further evidence as to a cause for the problem or problems. It may be appropriate to make referrals to other healthcare professionals such as: physiotherapists in order to assist the patient in removing respiratory tract secretions; the surgical team (e.g. if the patient develops an acute abdomen); or the radiologist for advice regarding specific imaging that may be helpful.

CONCLUSION

The use of an Early Warning System is becoming commonplace and is a useful tool to identify those patients at risk of deterioration. It has the potential to assist the healthcare practitioner in the care of the patient in that: it assists in prioritising those patients that need the greatest input in terms of observations, escalation in care, and referrals to other healthcare specialists such as the Critical Care Outreach Team. It meets the suggestions laid out in NICE Clinical Guideline 50 (NICE, 2007) in that it facilitates a graded response to patient need. For example, rather than a blanket strategy of all patients having observations done two to four hourly to detect potential deterioration, the EWS provides the healthcare practitioner with additional information to use in order to rationalise the care provided in the clinical environment. So, using EWS scores, it is possible to allocate some patients to have observations done twice a day and to designate those with higher scores, and therefore at greater risk of deterioration, to have their observations taken more frequently. Where EWS may increase workload for some it can be used to prioritise and reduce workload also. EWS is not a replacement for clinical judgement and can only be used to assist in this, nor is it a predictor of patient outcome. Using EWS correctly allows us to detect patients at risk of deterioration at an early stage; however, this is of little use if we do not communicate effectively and intervene in order to prevent the deterioration progressing.

There should be little doubt in the mind of the healthcare practitioner as to the benefits of an A to E assessment. Using this approach in the assessment of the acutely ill patient saves lives. It gives the healthcare professional a framework within which to act that ensures the greatest threats to life are detected and addressed early. In using this approach it is easier to remember the essential things to look at and in which order, intervening or referring to others as appropriate along the continuum of A to E, thereby reducing time wastage. The effect of this is prompt life-preserving treatment for the patient and increasing confidence for the healthcare professional that they can deal with this kind of scenario if it arises, as they have the necessary skills at their disposal.

SIMULATION SCENARIO

Introduction

A 64-year-old obese male admitted to the Orthopaedic trauma ward from the Emergency Department. Seven-day history of right-sided hip pain, swelling and redness, feels hot. You don't like the look of him; he has a high respiratory rate and a funny breathing pattern. Past medical history = arthritis affecting the right hip and obesity.

Table 3.4

Learning objectives	• Demonstrate safe, competent practice in a patient simulation situation encompassing skills A to E • Understand the rationale for using a systematic approach • Be able to discuss the A to E approach to patient assessment and each of its individual components • Discuss and evaluate the healthcare practitioner's application of the EWS and A to E approach during the scenario • Be able to calculate an Early Warning Score (EWS) based on local EWS chart
Resources	*Equipment* • Selection of airways, oral and naso-pharyngeal • Flow meters • Suction, yankeur and suction catheters • Selection of methods for administering oxygen • Stethoscope • Cannulas – assorted • Blood bottles – assorted • Blood culture bottles • Fluids – assorted • Fluid administration set • Catheter bag • Pen torch *Setting* • Clinical as possible • Hospital bed and linen • Simulated/real oxygen ports *People* • Candidate • Simulator/Facilitator – (can play patient's relative also) • Assistant *Time* • 45 mins including review of performance
Airway	• Oxygen should be applied immediately via 15L non-rebreathe mask • Patent and self-maintained (initially) • Occasional deep breaths with accompanied snoring sounds
Breathing	• Respiratory rate 12/min – erratic pattern. Stops for periods of approximately 15 seconds followed by a very deep breath. If shaken or painful stimuli – wakes and breathes normally for a short time then goes off to sleep again. Recurs through the whole scenario • $SpO_2 = 99\%$ on 10L O_2 via non-rebreathe mask. Blood gas shows Lactate 5.9 mmol/L, pO_2 12kPa, pCO_2 7.5kPA, pH 7.21 • On auscultation, good air entry throughout, nil added sounds

(Continued)

Table 3.4   (Continued)

Circulation	• BP 100/50, HR 115/min (regular), capillary refill time = 4 seconds, Temp 38.6°C. Nil antimicrobials prescribed. Blood results reveal raised urea, creatinine and potassium levels • Access 1x small cannula – tissued • No urinary catheter – Wife if asked states patient has not passed urine for at least 12 hours
Disability	• AVPU – variable, starts as **V** but as the examination progresses deteriorates to **P** – associated with apnoeic episodes. Pupils equal and responsive to light • Blood Sugar = 11.0mmol/L
Exposure	• Obese. Nil abdominal or calf tenderness • Right hip, scar present from previous total hip replacement • Right hip appears red and swollen, feels hot to the touch

The patient's wife has been present throughout and is very concerned.

The healthcare practitioner should be encouraged to assess the patient using the A to E approach; the facilitator will be required to give extra information throughout the scenario based on the actions of the healthcare practitioner. A calculation of the patient's EWS based on the observations provided should be undertaken, **but should not take place in preference/prior to instigating any emergency treatment.**

Roles of Participants

Facilitator – should present the information given in the introduction and ask the candidate to repeat it in order to assess retention of information. It should be specified that help can be given, but **only if requested**. Ensure the candidate works through the A to E assessment in the correct order and instigates treatment appropriately. Correct, safe practice adhering to local protocols and infection control should be demonstrated throughout, e.g. including correct sizing of airways. Be reactive to actions of the candidate – e.g. fluid cannot be given until additional access is secured. If a bag of fluid is given there should be no immediate improvement and the candidate should be encouraged to repeat this action – in order to support this decision they should be encouraged to look for signs of overload – none will be present so further fluid administration would be appropriate. If the candidate attempts to refer to a different team for them to take over straightaway, they should be informed that this will not occur for some time and they should proceed with their assessment.

Wife – can also be played by facilitator and if asked should only give information supporting that in the introduction, but also volunteers that she doesn't feel the patient has been to pass urine in at least 12 hours and was complaining of thirst for two days prior to admission and that he was getting 'very sweaty' and 'shivering'.

Assistant – available if requested – should be helpful and able to cannulate, take blood and catheterise if requested to do so. Should be guided by the candidate.

Human patient simulator – lies in bed, takes on the respiratory characteristics as described. Drowsy and doesn't respond unless painful stimuli applied, then only stays awake for a short period. If the candidate considers placing an airway, they should describe correct technique – the patient would gag on an oral airway, but tolerate a nasopharyngeal airway once inserted. If questioned in one of the more awake phases the patient should describe pain in the right hip, feeling exhausted, feeling shivery despite having pyrexia, and being extremely thirsty. The patient is relatively passive throughout the scenario.

Points for discussion

At the end of the scenario candidates should work out the EWS on the initial observations and discuss the role of this and the A to E assessment in the examination of the deteriorating/acutely unwell individual. They should be encouraged to think about potential differential diagnoses and what escalation may be required including specialist help, further examinations or transfer to another area. They should also be prompted to discuss what they felt went well and if they would do anything differently if facing a similar scenario again. This scenario could be enhanced if there is the facility to video record the scenario and play it back to the candidates to aid debrief.

REFERENCES

British National Formulary (2009) *Joint Formulary Committee*. London: BMJ group and RPS publishing.

Cretikos, M.A., Bellomo, R., Hillman, K., Chen, J., Finfer, S. and Flabouris, A. (2008) 'Respiratory rate: the neglected vital sign', *The Medical Journal of Australia*, 188 (11): 657–9.

Kumar, A., Roberts, D., Wood, K.E., Light, B., Parrillo, J.E., Sharma, S., Suppes, R., Feinstein, D., Zanotti, S. and Taiberg, L. (2006) 'Duration of hypotension before initiation of effective antimicrobial therapy is the critical determinant of survival in human septic shock', *Critical Care Medicine*, 34: 1589–96.

Mallett, J. and Dougherty, L. (eds) (2001) *The Royal Marsden Manual of Clinical Nursing Procedures*, 5th edn. Oxford: Blackwell Science.

National Institute for Health and Clinical Excellence (NICE) (2007) *Acutely Ill Patients in Hospital. Recognition of and Response to Acute Illness in Adults in Hospital*. London: NICE. Available on: http://www.nice.org.uk/nicemedia/pdf/CG50FullGuidance.pdf [accessed 21 January 2011].

Nolan, J. et al. (eds) (2008) *Advanced Life Support Course Manual*, 5th edn. London: Resuscitation Council (UK).

Simpson, P. (Chairman) (2005) *An Acute Problem?* London: NCEPOD. Available on: http://www.ncepod.org.uk/2005report/summary.pdf [accessed 21 January 2011].

Smith, G.B. (2003a) *Acute Life Threatening Event Recognition and Treatment Course Handbook*, 2nd edn. University Of Portsmouth: Learning Media Development.

Smith, G.B. (2003b) *ALERT Course Manual*. Project Report. University of Portsmouth Press.

UHL Surgical Early Warning System reproduced with permission of UHL and designer C. Barclay Critical Care Outreach Lead.

Walker, H.K., Hall, W.D. and Hurst, J.W. (eds) (1990) *Clinical Methods: The History, Physical and Laboratory Examinations*, 3rd edn. Boston: Butterworths. Available on: http://www.ncbi.nlm.nih.gov/books/NBK420/ [accessed 21 January 2011].

4

OBSERVATIONS: BLOOD PRESSURE, PULSE/HEART RATE, TEMPERATURE AND NEUROLOGICAL ASSESSMENT

Chris Jones

Aim

The aim of this chapter is to discuss the importance of vital signs observation in healthcare practice.

Objectives

The healthcare professional will:

- Be able to discuss the importance of vital signs measurement.
- Be able to discuss the technique for respiratory rate measurement.
- Be able to the technique for discuss blood pressure measurement.
- Be able to discuss the technique for temperature measurement.
- Be able to discuss the technique for pulse/heart rate measurement.
- Be able to discuss conscious level assessment.

BOX 4.1: VITAL SIGNS

- Respiratory rate
- Pulse/heart rate
- Blood pressure
- Temperature
- Conscious level assessment

The need for healthcare professionals being able to carry out vital sign observations competently, accurately interpret the data and make appropriate decisions is a key factor in reducing the number of unnecessary deaths, reducing hospital stay and the cost of treatment.

The National Patient Safety Agency (2007) analysed patient safety incident forms from 2005; of the 64 incidents related to a patient death, three common themes emerged:

1 Failure to measure basic observations of vital signs
2 A lack of recognition of the importance of worsening vital signs
3 A delay in responding to deteriorating vital signs.

Recognising deterioration in a critically ill patient not only reduces the risk of cardiopulmonary arrest but also has implications for length of treatment, hospital stay and cost of treatment. As The National Patient Safety Agency (2007: 16) states: 'Patients whose deterioration is not picked up early, but who do not proceed to cardiac arrest, will also have increased avoidable morbidity, increased length of stay and associated avoidable healthcare costs'.

The monitoring of vital signs is not just important to detect deterioration, but to also establish a baseline for patient assessment during the patient journey and to assist with clinical diagnosis in a number of conditions (e.g. shock, worsening head injuries).

As a skill that may be required to be performed in a number of settings by a variety of healthcare professionals, a **comprehensive understanding of the procedures is vital** when performing, monitoring and reporting vital signs.

VITAL SIGN ASSESSMENT

Segen (2006: 736) defines a vital sign as: 'Any objective parameter used to assess basic life functions – e.g., Blood Pressure (BP), pulse, respiratory rate, and temperature'.

This chapter will concentrate on the vital signs that the National Institute for Health and Clinical Excellence (NICE) (2007a) advocate should be recorded as an initial assessment and as part of routine monitoring in an acute hospital setting. These are:

- Respiratory assessment
- Pulse/heart rate
- Blood pressure
- Temperature
- Conscious level

PREPARATION AS A SKILL

When undertaking any procedure the healthcare professional should pay particular attention to preparing themselves, their patient, the environment and equipment. This process should include:

- Ensuring the patient is in an appropriate area for assessment; the area should be private, warm, and have oxygen, suction and monitoring nearby
- Introducing yourself and your role
- Ensuring the right patient is having the correct observation performed
- Explaining to the patient what vital sign is going to be assessed and how it is going to be undertaken
- Gaining consent before proceeding
- Washing hands before and after contact with a patient.

By performing these actions the professional will:

- Reduce anxiety
- Maintain patient safety
- Maintain the patient's comfort, privacy and dignity
- Ensure the patient understands and has given consent for the observation to be performed
- Prevent the spread of infection.

RESPIRATORY ASSESSMENT

DEFINITION OF RESPIRATORY RATE AND PATTERN

Normal ventilation is an automatic, seemingly effortless inspiratory expansion and expiratory contraction of the chest cage. This act of normal breathing has a relatively constant rate and inspiratory volume that together constitute normal respiratory rhythm. The accessory muscles of inspiration (sternocleidomastoid and scalenes) and expiration (abdominal) are not normally used in the resting state. Abnormalities may occur in rate, rhythm, and in the effort of breathing. (Braun, 1990: 226)

Deterioration in respiratory function is one of the major causes of critical illness in the United Kingdom (NICE, 2007a). Considine (2005) states there is a link between respiratory dysfunction, critical illness and eventual mortality.

PRIOR KNOWLEDGE NEEDED TO EFFECTIVELY PERFORM A RESPIRATORY OBSERVATION

- The anatomy and physiology of the respiratory and cardiovascular systems
- The physiological process of respiration
- How common respiratory diseases affect respiratory function
- Normal values for adults.

ASSESSING RESPIRATION – PROCEDURE

Table 4.1

Action	Rationale
Wherever possible ask patient to undress and give theatre gown	To visualise the chest and identify signs of respiratory distress
Commence assessment	
Look at:	
Patient's position	To identify discomfort due to respiratory distress (e.g. unable to lie flat, sitting in an upright position)
Signs of respiratory distress	To identify use of accessory muscles suggesting respiratory distress
Respiratory rate; one respiration consists of an inspiration and expiration	To detect for early signs of deterioration
Pattern and depth; chest movement should be symmetrical	To identify factors that may affect rate such as hypoxia and pain
Count rate for one full minute	To account for any irregular breathing in pattern/rate
Listen for:	
Breath sounds	Normal breathing is quiet; noisy breathing may indicate underlying problem, e.g. asthma suggested by wheeze, stridor may indicate epiglottitis
If abnormal rate or signs of respiratory distress report finding *immediately* to a senior member of staff; assist with instigating emergency procedures	Early treatment reduces the risk of poor prognosis

DISCUSSION POINTS

- How can patient history and factors such as smoking, obesity and medical past history affect findings?
- Respiratory rate will change if the patient is aware the rate is being assessed. What methods could be employed to overcome this?

PULSE/HEART RATE RECORDING

DEFINITION

The pulse is a Pressure wave that is transmitted through the arterial tree with each heart beat following the expansion and recoil of arteries during each cardiac cycle. A pulse can be palpated in any artery that lies close to the surface of the body. (Marieb and Hoehn, 2007, cited in Dougherty and Lister, 2008: 497)

Traditionally, pulse measurement has been considered as one of the four vital signs of life (Endacott et al., 2009) as it is a fundamental indication of health status. The presence of a pulse indicates the heart is able sufficiently to pump blood around the body to perfuse tissue; changes in pulse rate may be an early indication of deterioration of a patient's condition.

PRIOR KNOWLEDGE NEEDED EFFECTIVELY TO PERFORM A PULSE OBSERVATION

- Anatomy and physiology of the cardiovascular system
- The process involved in the cardiac cycle
- Symptoms of illness/injuries that may affect pulse rate/character
- Terminology required to describe pulse character (e.g. weak, bounding, etc.)
- Medical terminology (e.g. tachycardia/bradycardia)
- Normal parameters of pulse rate
- The common sites for pulse recording.

MEASURING A RADIAL/BRACHIAL PULSE PROCEDURE

Practice such as measuring for 30 seconds then multiplying by two should not be encouraged, as this does not take account of irregularities in beat.

Table 4.2

Action	Rationale
Ensure patient is sitting comfortably with arm well supported	To minimise discomfort

Assessment
• Locate the pulse that you wish to assess
   o *Radial*: same side on the wrist as the thumb (see Figure 4.1)
   o *Brachial*: ante cubital fossa follow along the line of the small finger met acarpal
	To be able to palpate the blood passing through the artery, without occluding the artery

• When pulse is found using the pads of the second and third fingers, press gently, but do not press too hard • Using the second hand of a watch measure the pulse for one minute; note pulse rate, character and volume	To ensure factors such as irregularity are considered in pulse measurement

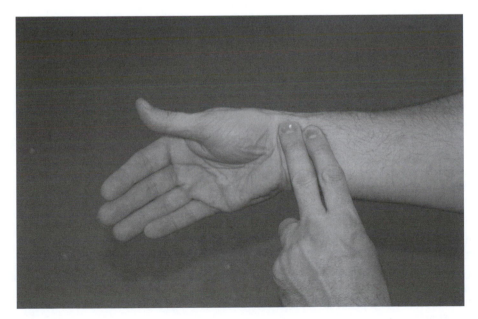

Figure 4.1

BLOOD PRESSURE

DEFINITION OF BLOOD PRESSURE

Blood Pressure is the pressure exerted on the wall of blood vessels by the blood inside them. (Endacott et al., 2009: 212)

Measuring blood pressure will help to evaluate the effectiveness of the cardiovascular system. Changes in blood pressure can indicate problems with cardiovascular status and can provide subtle clues to deterioration in a patient's condition.

PRIOR KNOWLEDGE REQUIRED TO PERFORM A BLOOD PRESSURE MEASUREMENT EFFECTIVELY

- Anatomy and physiology of the cardiovascular system
- The mechanism of blood pressure
- The cardiac cycle
- Common cardiac conditions that may influence blood pressure
- How to palpate the radial and brachial pulse
- Common medical terminology
- Indications for measuring blood pressure.

STEP-BY-STEP PROCEDURE – MERCURY/ANEROID SPHYGMOMANOMETER

Table 4.3

Action	Rationale
Ensure patient is in an appropriate quiet area for assessment	To be able to listen for Korotkoff sounds
Check with patient any contra-indications to using a particular limb to measure blood pressure	To reduce distress and risk of causing unnecessary pain
Ensure patient's legs uncrossed	To reduce risk of abnormal results
Ensure there are no tight garments around the upper arm	To gain access to upper arm and ensure stethoscope head is placed correctly
Guide the patient's arm into the correct supported position – level with heart and use a pillow to support arm	Ensures accurate measurement

Table 4.4

Action	Rationale
Prepare equipment	
• Ensure sphygmomanometer has been checked for safety and recently serviced	To reduce risk of error
• Ensure all equipment clean and intact	To reduce cross infection and risk of abnormal reading
• Ensure sphygmomanometer on a level surface at eye level	To maintain good posture and enable easy interpretation of reading
• Ensure you have a wide range of cuff sizes	A wrongly sized bladder may lead to under or overestimation of blood pressure
• Measure cuff to cover 80% of arm circumference	Too large bladder will restrict stethoscope access to the brachial artery
• Ensure stethoscope is clean; place earpiece in ears and tap the diaphragm	To reduce impediment to hearing Korotkoff sounds
Procedure	
• Locate the brachial pulse	To enable cuff and stethoscope application
• Apply the cuff firmly to arm ensuring the artery marker is two fingerbreadth above the brachial artery (see Figure 4.2)	To reduce bladder movement and ensure cuff is in correct position for occluding the brachial artery; reduces noise interference when listening for Korotkoff sounds
• Ask patient not to speak while measuring blood pressure	Speaking can raise blood pressure and distract practitioner from listening to Korotkoff sounds
• Place stethoscope in ears ensuring head of stethoscope nearby	To ensure quick placement of stethoscope head when ready to deflate cuff
• While palpating brachial pulse inflate the cuff; observe the mercury column/dial as cuff inflates, note the reading when you cannot feel the pulse	To estimate systolic blood pressure
• Insert earpieces of stethoscope and place the bell of the stethoscope over the brachial pulse point; re-inflate the cuff up to 20–30mmHg above your estimated systolic blood pressure	

(Continued)

Table 4.4 (Continued)

Action	Rationale
• Open valve to deflate cuff slowly, aiming for mercury/dial to drop 2mmHg per second. Watch the dial/mercury closely	To auscultate Korotkoff sounds
• When you hear the first two consecutive taps of Korotkoff sounds, note the point of the mercury/dial	To obtain a reading of the systolic blood pressure
• As the cuff deflates listen for when the Korotkoff sounds disappear, note the point of the mercury/dial	To obtain a reading of the diastolic blood pressure
• Allow the cuff to deflate completely until 20mmHg below the diastolic pressure has been reached	To minimise the risk of a false reading
• Remove cuff from patient's arm	
• Record measurement on appropriate observation chart/ early warning system, clearly recording date, time and arm or limb used. Consider documenting whether patient sitting or lying during measurement	To provide a written record of observation
• Clean stethoscope earpieces according to trust policy	To reduce cross infection

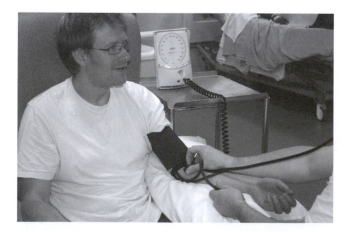

Figure 4.2

DISCUSSION POINTS

Automated Blood Pressure vs Manual Blood Pressure

O'Brien et al. (2003) describe manual blood pressure as the 'Gold standard of blood pressure measurement'. Manual blood pressure appears to be disappearing from clinical practice and the use of automated machines has become more common. Automatic blood pressure monitors can be useful, but as a baseline measurement and in critically ill patients, manual blood pressure measurement should be considered.

Table 4.5 discusses briefly some of the advantages and disadvantages of manual/automatic blood pressure monitoring as suggested by O'Brien et al. (2003). It is up to the individual practitioner and local policy to decide on which method to adopt when measuring blood pressure.

Table 4.5

	Advantages	Disadvantages
Manual BP	Reliable	Technique needs to be precise
	Equipment easily checked and maintained	Can increase blood pressure through 'white coat syndrome'
		Repeated use of equipment can lead to inaccuracy in reading
Automatic	Needs less intensive training to perform	Results have been found to be inaccurate
	Can store trends and findings	Cannot record blood pressure in all circumstances (e.g. atrial fibrillation)
	Easy to interpret	

TEMPERATURE MEASUREMENT

DEFINITION OF TEMPERATURE

Body Temperature represents the balance between heat gain and heat loss. (Marieb and Hoehn, 2007, cited in Dougherty and Lister, 2008: 522)

Temperature is an important measurement to perform as it can provide an indication of minor/major illnesses. These may include:

- Sepsis
- Reaction to blood transfusion
- Infection.

KNOWLEDGE REQUIRED PRIOR TO COMMENCING THIS PROCEDURE

- Normal temperature values
- Anatomy and physiology of skin and its relation to temperature control

- Temperature regulation
- Accepted sites for temperature monitoring
- Terminology used to describe temperature (hypothermia, pyrexia)
- Types of temperature recording equipment available and indication for use
- Conditions where a patient's temperature requires careful monitoring.

TEMPERATURE – PROCEDURE

DISCUSSION POINTS

- The importance of correct thermometer placement in obtaining an accurate reading.
- Factors that may lead to an inaccurate reading in tympanic measurement.
- Criteria for choosing route to record temperature (e.g. axilla temperature should not be the chosen site of recording for the patient with suspected hypothermia).
- Rectal temperatures are now not advocated due to its invasive nature; however, in certain conditions where an accurate core temperature is required, such as in hypothermia, this route should be considered (Lefrant et al., 2003).

CONSCIOUS LEVEL ASSESSMENT

DEFINITION

Consciousness is defined as the state of being aware of physical events or mental concepts. Conscious patients are awake and responsive to their surroundings. (Marcovitch, 2005: 158)

The conscious level is important as decreased conscious level can affect the functioning of other systems (NICE, 2007a). Therefore, early recognition of deteriorating conscious level is vital to support the maintenance of airway, breathing and circulation.

KNOWLEDGE REQUIRED PRIOR TO UNDERTAKING THIS PROCEDURE

- Causes of decreased conscious level
- Effects of altered conscious level in managing airway, breathing and circulation
- Anatomy and physiology of the nervous system
- Medical terminology (e.g. decorticate posture)
- National recommendations and trust policy regarding frequency of observations.

Table 4.6

Action	Rationale
Axilla Temperature Measurement	
• Check patient has not had a recent hot bath, fluids or engaged in exercise	These factors may cause a temporary rise in temperature
• Remove clothing to expose one axilla	To ensure thermometer placed in correct position
• Ensure skin of axilla clean and dry	Moisture between skin of an axilla could affect reading
• If using electronic thermometer, ensure clean cover in situ and is in working order; ensure thermometer set to axilla mode	To reduce risk of cross infection and reduce risk of error caused by faulty equipment/setting
• Place thermometer in axilla surrounded by skin surfaces	
• Place patient's arm across chest	To reduce risk of inaccurate reading caused by incorrect placement or thermometer movement
• Leave thermometer under axilla for amount of time advocated by manufacturer	
• When appropriate time reached remove thermometer and read temperature measured	To monitor temperature
Oral Temperature Measurement	
• Consider factors that may affect readings o hot/cold drinks o oxygen therapy o smoking	This will temporarily affect reading and you may need to consider other sites
• If using electronic thermometer ensure clean cover in situ and is in working order; ensure thermometer set to oral mode	To reduce risk of cross infection and reduce risk of error caused by faulty equipment/setting
• Place thermometer in either left or right hand side at junction of floor of the mouth and base of tongue	To reduce risk of inaccurate reading caused by incorrect placement
• Ask patient to keep mouth closed	To minimise risk of error caused by air through the mouth
• Leave thermometer under oral cavity for amount of time advocated by manufacturer	To ensure accurate technique employed
• When appropriate time reached remove thermometer and read temperature measured	To monitor temperature

(Continued)

Table 4.6   (Continued)

Action	Rationale
Rectal Temperature	

• Consider contraindications to using site
   ○ *rectal surgery*
   ○ *haemorrhoids*	

• Wash hands and apply non sterile gloves	
• Lie patient on left hand side with knees bent	To minimise distress and provide easy access to rectum
• If using electronic thermometer ensure clean cover in situ and is in working order; ensure thermometer set to rectal mode	To reduce risk of cross infection and reduce risk of error caused by faulty equipment/setting
• Lubricate thermometer probe prior to insertion	To minimise distress and ease insertion, minimise risk of mucosal damage
• Gently insert probe 2–4cm and hold in position for required time	To reduce risk of inaccurate reading caused by incorrect placement/movement
• After required time remove probe, dispose with gloves, and record temperature	To reduce risk of cross infection
Tympanic Measurement	

• Consider factors that may affect readings:
   ○ Ear wax
   ○ Otitis externa/media
   ○ Lying on side with ear to be measured against a pillow prior to procedure
   ○ Ear hair
   ○ Hearing aids
	These factors will provide an inaccurate reading, therefore consider other sites or attempting measurement at a later time.

• Assist patient in maintaining a comfortable position	To allow easy access to ear canal
• If indicated switch thermometer on	To ensure thermometer ready for use
• Using sleeve box, apply disposable thermometer cover without touching with fingers	
• Gently pull the earlobe upwards and insert the thermometer until it snugly fits into the ear canal, sealing the opening	Reduce cross infection To reduce risk of cover wrinkling, leading to inaccurate measurement To safely introduce thermometer, straighten the ear canal and position probe for accurate view of tympanic membrane, thus reducing risk of interference from ambient air temperature
• Measure the temperature according to manufacturer's instructions	
• Remove probe, dispose of cover in clinical waste	

AVPU

AVPU assessment is a quick and easy way to assess conscious level. It was initially taught as part of the Advanced Trauma and Life Support Course, but has now been incorporated into early warning scores. AVPU assesses the patient response using the following criteria.

Alert
Voice
Pain
Unresponsive

ASSESSING CONSCIOUS LEVEL USING AVPU – PROCEDURE

Table 4.7

Action	Rationale
Assess: Airway Breathing Circulation	To ensure patient airway and instigate early emergency treatment
As you approach patient note if they have their eyes open prior to speaking to them	If patient's eyes are open prior to speaking they are *Alert*, if they are closed then assess response to speech
If the patient's eyes are closed firmly ask an implicit question (e.g. can you open your eyes?)	If the patient opens their eyes they are *responding to speech*. If no response, then assess response to pain
Using the thumb and two fingers, hold the trapezius muscle where the neck meets the shoulder and squeeze	If the patient responds they are *responding to pain*, if there is no response they are unresponsive

N.B. *If patient unresponsive then the student should state they would instigate emergency procedures:*

- *Call for help/support*
- *Airway management as appropriate*

GLASGOW COMA SCORE

The National Institute for Health and Clinical Excellence (NICE, 2007b) recommend the use of the Glasgow Coma Score (GCS) as required documentation when performing observation of the patient with a neurological injury/illness.

GLASGOW COMA SCORE – PROCEDURE

Table 4.8

Action	Rationale
Assess: Airway Breathing Circulation	To ensure patient airway and instigate early emergency treatment
Eye Opening (E)	
As you approach patient, note if they have their eyes open prior to you speaking to them	If patient's eyes are open prior to you speaking they are *Alert and the score will be four.* If they are closed then assess response to speech
If the patient's eyes are closed firmly ask a direct question (e.g. can you open your eyes?)	If the patient opens their eyes, they are *responding to speech and the score will be three.* If no response, then assess response to pain
Using the thumb and two fingers, hold the trapezius muscle where the neck meets the shoulder and squeeze	If the patient responds they are *responding to pain and the score will be two.* If there is no response, they are *unresponsive and the score is one*
Verbal Response (V)	
Ask patient simple clear questions (e.g. what is your name, where are you? What is the date?)	To assess verbal response If able to answer coherently *the score is five*
Note patient response, listening for:	
• Confused conversation	If the patient is confused, while being able to answer they will not be able to answer correctly one or more of these questions, therefore *the score is four*
• The patient using inappropriate words to reply	*Score is three*
• If the patient replies but is incomprehensible (e.g. moans, grunts)	*Score is two*
• No response	*Score is one*
Best Motor Response (M)	
If the patient is alert or responding to voice ask the patient to do something (e.g. Can you squeeze my fingers?)	If the patient does what you ask, their *score is six*

(Continued)

Table 4.8   *(Continued)*

Action	Rationale
If there is no response to voice, perform a trapezium squeeze and look for response. If the patient:	
• Localises where the pain is and tries to push you away	*Score five*
• Withdraws	*Score four*
• Adopts a decorticate posture	*Score three*
• Adopts a decerebrate position	*Score two*
• If there is no response	*Score one*
Add together the scores found for eye opening, motor and verbal response to get a total score (e.g. E = four, V = five, M = six. Total score = 15) The minimum score will be three, maximum is 15	To evaluate conscious level
Assess pupils for:	
• Size (compare with guide on neurological chart)	Both pupils should be equal size, but size may be affected by certain illness/injury
• Reaction to light. With the room darkened bring the light from one side and shine directly into eye; both pupils should constrict. There should be a consensual reaction, i.e. right eye should also constrict when light shined into left eye	Abnormal pupil reaction may be a sign of underlying brain dysfunction caused by illness/injury

Please note: a GCS score of less than nine is consistent with a coma and will require advanced airway management.

DISCUSSION POINTS

Patient Problems Affecting Understanding of GCS

• Hard of hearing/deafness
• Language barriers
• Learning disabilities.

(Continued)

(Continued)

How to Overcome these Problems

- Checking for hearing aids
- Using simple language/questions to reduce risk of misunderstanding
- Position self in patient's field of vision
- Family involvement in patients with learning disabilities
- Techniques used to determine response to pain
- Advantages and disadvantages of AVPU/GCS

After finishing any vital sign observations, it is the healthcare professional's responsibility to:

- Record findings on an appropriate observation/early warning system chart
- Compare observations found with previous recordings
- Be aware of trends suggesting improvement/deterioration in condition
- Report any abnormal findings to relevant professionals and instigate urgent treatment if indicated
- Store equipment away safely.

CONCLUSION

Measuring vital signs, although frequently performed, is often dismissed as a basic skill; however, actually performing these observations requires considerable skill and provides a number of challenges professionally, legally and ethically.

When performing these observations the professional has a duty of care to make their patient comfortable, maintain their privacy and dignity, and instigate treatment based on findings. Poor technique and interpretation can lead to longer treatment, increased length of stay, higher cost of treatment and – in extreme circumstances – a preventable death.

Therefore, the training of professionals in these skills is of the upmost importance. Utilising simulation enables the healthcare student to understand the process behind a skill. Simulation also enables the student professional to practise in a safe, protected environment free of potential patient harm/litigation.

SIMULATION SCENARIO

Vital Sign Assessment Skills

Learning Outcomes

The following are **possible** learning outcomes that the student could achieve.

General Skills

By using simulation the student should be able to:

- Identify interpersonal skills required when performing vital sign assessment, and the importance of safe practice

- Demonstrate skills required to keep the patient warm, comfortable and maintain their privacy and dignity
- Interpret observations to recognise abnormal results and instigate emergency treatment
- Recognise the importance of team work and leadership in professional practice
- Record findings on a observation chart
- Demonstrate awareness of infection control procedures
- Identify the procedure to take if values are abnormal or emergency procedures required.

Respiratory Assessment Skills

By using simulation the student should be able to:

- Understand the importance of respiratory assessment
- Establish the skills required to perform a full respiratory assessment
- Show awareness of normal respiratory rates in adult patients
- Demonstrate and practise observational skills.

Pulse Assessment Skills

By using simulation the student should be able to:

- Identify and accurately locate the site of major pulse points in the body
- Demonstrate knowledge of the normal pulse rates in adult patients.

Blood Pressure Skills

By using simulation the student should be able to:

- Demonstrate knowledge of the importance of blood pressure measurement
- Demonstrate knowledge of normal values in an adult patient
- Demonstrate skills required to perform a blood pressure measurement
- Demonstrate the importance of cleaning and checking equipment prior to use
- Demonstrate and practise observational skills
- Discuss the limitations of using automated devices to record blood pressure.

Temperature Measurement

By using simulation the student should be able to:

- Provide a rationale for the chosen site of measurement
- Measure temperature using a variety of equipment.

Assessing Conscious Level

By using simulation the student should be:

- Aware of conscious level assessment in ABCDE assessment
- Aware of the procedure to assess conscious level
- Aware of the different tools used to assess conscious level.

Simulation Teaching Resources Required

Equipment

- Watch with a second hand
- Observation/early warning chart and pen
- Cleaning equipment
- Stethoscope
- Pillows
- Sphygmomanometer
- Blood pressure cuff, various sizes
- Appropriate thermometer, e.g.
  - Disposable
  - Tympanic and probe covers
  - Electronic thermometer and cover
- Gloves
- Pen torch
- For this scenario the use of a role player as a patient or a simulation manikin with set parameters would be acceptable.

Setting

In this scenario the ideal setting could be a ward setting/GP Surgery.

Timing

In this example for a three-hour session you may need:

- Introduction and aims (10 minutes)
- Skills procedure – respiratory assessment (10 minutes)
- Feedback (5 minutes)
- Pulse assessment (10 minutes)
- Feedback (5 minutes)
- Blood pressure (10 minutes)
- Feedback (5 minutes)
- Temperature (10 minutes)
- Feedback (5 minutes)
- Conscious level (20 minutes)
- Debrief and discussion (30 minutes)

Timing should be adaptable.

Scenario

- Should encourage a structured holistic assessment
- Should be clear on what you want the student to do.

In this example the scenario could be:
Joe Evans is an 86-year-old man who has presented to the emergency department following a collapse. You have been asked by your mentor to go and assess his vital signs.

Roles of Participants

Mentor – Role should be taken by facilitator
Student – Role should be taken by student healthcare professional (may be more than one to encourage team working)
Other members of group should participate in observing and giving feedback to student.

Points for Debrief

- Obtaining consent
- Technique used to measure observation
- Did the student(s) maintain privacy, dignity and maintain comfort? Was it safe practice?
- Interpreting results
- Did the student accurately interpret the results and escalate care accordingly?
- Documentation
- Document effectively using appropriate chart?

REFERENCES

Braun, S. (1990) 'Respiratory rate and pattern', in: H.K. Walker, W.D. Hall and J.W. Hurst (1990) *Clinical Methods: The History, Physical, and Laboratory Examinations*, 3rd edn. Boston: Butterworths.

Braun, S., Walker, H.K., Hall, W.D. and Hurst, J.W. (1990) *Clinical Methods: The History, Physical, and Laboratory Examinations*, 3rd edn. Boston: Butterworths.

Considine, J. (2005) 'The role of nurses in preventing adverse events related to respiratory dysfunction: literature review', *Journal of Advanced Nursing*, 49 (6): 624–33.

Dougherty, L. and Lister, S. (2008) *The Royal Marsden Hospital Manual of Clinical Nursing Procedures*, 7th edn. Chichester: Wiley-Blackwell.

Endacott, R., Jevon, P. and Cooper, S. (2009) *Clinical Nursing Skills Core and Advanced*. Oxford: Oxford University Press.

Lefrant, J.Y., Muller, L., Emmanuel Coussaye, J., Benbabaali, M., Lebris, C., Zeitoun, N., Mari, C., Saissi, G., Ripart, J. and Eledjam, J.J. (2003) 'Temperature measurement in intensive care patients: comparison of urinary bladder, oesophageal, rectal, axillary, and inguinal methods versus pulmonary artery core method', *Intensive Care Medicine*, 29 (33): 414–18.

MacLellan, K. (2004) 'Postoperative pain: strategy for improving patients' experiences: issues and interventions in nursing practice', *Journal of Advanced Nursing*, 46 (2): 179–85.

Marcovitch, H. (2005) *Black's Medical Dictionary*. London: Black.

Marieb, E. and Hoehn, K. (2007) 'Human anatomy and physiology', in L. Dougherty and S. Lister (2008) *The Royal Marsden Hospital Manual of Clinical Nursing Procedures*, 7th edn. Chichester: Wiley-Blackwell.

National Institute for Health and Clinical Excellence (NICE) (2007a) *Acutely Ill Patients in Hospital. Recognition of and Response to Acute Illness in Adults in Hospital*. London: NICE.

National Institute for Health and Clinical Excellence (NICE) (2007b) *Head Injury: Triage, Assessment, Investigation and Early Management of Head Injury in Infants, Children and Adults*. London: NICE.

National Patient Safety Agency (NPSA) (2007) *The Fifth Report from the Patient Safety Observatory. Safer Care for the Acutely Ill Patient: Learning From Serious Incidents*. London: NPSA.

O'Brien, E., Asmar, R., Beilin, L., Imai, Y., Mallion, J.-M., Mancia, G., Mengden, T., Myers, M., Padfield, P., Palatini, P., Parati, G., Pickering, T., Redon, J., Staessen, J., Stergiou, G. and Verdecchia, P. (2003) 'European Society of Hypertension recommendations for conventional, ambulatory and home blood pressure measurement', *Journal of Hypertension*, 21: 821–48.

Segen, J.C. (2006) *Concise Dictionary of Modern Medicine*, 2nd revd edn. New York: McGraw-Hill Professional.

5

PAIN ASSESSMENT

Meriel Hawker

Aim

The aim of this chapter is to equip the reader with the knowledge required to undertake effective pain assessment for their patients.

Objectives

On completion of this chapter the reader will be able to:

- Discuss and recognise the importance of undertaking pain assessment
- Describe the effects on the patient of under-treated pain
- Identify instances when pain assessment should be performed
- Practise the skill of assessing pain.

INTRODUCTION

For many people pain is a part of everyday life, for others it is a fleeting encounter. Its effects can be long lasting and life changing.

The International Association for the Study of Pain Montreal Declaration (IASP) (2010) states that it is 'the right of all people to have access to pain management without discrimination'; however, evidence suggests that frequently the management of pain is inadequate and often flawed (Sjöström et al., 2000). Evidence shows that pain is improperly addressed despite being a particular concern for patients

(Healthcare Commission, 2006). Studies have demonstrated that nurses extensively misjudge the intensity of patients' pain and often believe that patients may be exaggerating their pain (Sloman et al., 2005).

In general, nurses underestimate severe pain and overestimate mild pain. Sloman et al. (2005) go on to suggest that patients draw on their personal experiences of actually feeling pain, while nurses may relate to pain by unconsciously drawing on their clinical experiences of the multitude of patients they have cared for over the years. This may lead to disparity in pain management, with patients' reports of pain not matching nurses' expectations. Patients often believe that health professionals are more knowledgeable with regard to what is best for managing their pain. However, poor clinical practice in assessment of pain has been identified as the most significant factor in the failure of analgesia, particularly in acute pain (Dihle et al., 2006).

Assessment of pain is an important skill to accomplish. It is the first step towards managing an individual's pain and without accurate assessment effective pain management is impossible. Burglass (2007) agrees that accurate pain assessment is essential for successful pain management. Assessment is required to identify the nature of the pain, the individual characteristics of the pain, or to gauge the effectiveness of any pain management interventions (Sjöström et al., 2000). Bell and Duffy (2009) suggest that it is unethical and unprofessional to allow a patient to suffer unnecessary pain.

BACKGROUND

Pain is a sensation many of us will have encountered, however, our perceptions and experiences will vary greatly. In our role as a healthcare professional, many of our patients will also experience pain and each will interpret its meaning and significance differently. Try to think of how you would explain what pain is to someone who has never experienced pain before. It is not an easy thing to explain. It is difficult for us to explain our own pain, so trying to understand someone else's pain and responding accordingly is challenging.

Defining pain is problematical and there have been numerous definitions over the years. The IASP suggest that pain is 'an unpleasant sensory and emotional experience associated with actual or potential tissue damage, or described in terms of such damage' (Merskey and Bogduk, 1994: 210), with McCaffery (1979) implying that pain is 'whatever the experiencing person says it is, existing wherever they say it does'.

Each of these definitions highlights a different aspect of pain, but neither is all-encompassing. These definitions intimate that pain is a complex phenomenon and that the patient is the expert with regard to it. It is important to remember that pain is subjective; it is only known to the person experiencing it and there is no medical test that can establish whether or not a person is experiencing pain. All these complexities do not make pain assessment an easy skill to master.

TYPES OF PAIN

Specific terminology is used when describing different types of pain.

- **Nociceptive Pain** is caused when nerve receptors, known as nociceptors, are activated by noxious stimulus. This stimulus can be caused by tissue damage, infection, heat, cold or chemical irritant
- **Neuropathic Pain** is caused by a fault in the central or peripheral nervous system. It can be due to direct injury to the nerve, such as the case of sciatica where a vertebral disc may have compressed the nerve, or due to disease, such as shingles where the virus damages the nerves.

Pain can also be described as somatic or visceral.

- **Somatic Pain** refers to pain felt in the skin, muscles, bones, tendons, etc. Somatic pain can be described as superficial or deep. Superficial somatic pain is easier to locate. Pain from the skin is often referred to as superficial somatic pain. This is due to the large number of nociceptors found in the skin. Deep somatic pain may be pain from muscles. There are fewer nociceptors and, therefore, it is harder to describe accurately or pinpoint where the pain is originating from
- **Visceral pain** is felt in the internal organs and is the hardest to accurately isolate as there are very few nociceptors in the internal organs.

Pain assessment can be in relation to acute, chronic or cancer pain, or to a combination of some or all of these elements. Having an understanding of the different types of pain can aid in the assessment. Also, different types of pain may result in different intervention strategies.

ACUTE PAIN

'Acute pain is associated with acute injury or disease' (Royal College of Anaesthetists, 2003). It is seen to have a protective function and alert us to the possibility that something is wrong such as traumatic injury, surgery or infection. Acute pain usually has a rapid onset and a short duration. Once the tissue damage subsides then the pain typically settles.

CHRONIC PAIN

Chronic pain has been defined as

> Pain that either persists beyond the point that healing would be expected to be complete (usually taken to be 3–6 months) or that occurs in disease processes in which healing does not take place. The pain may be continuous or intermittent. Chronic pain can be experienced by those who do not have evidence of tissue damage. (International Association for the Study of Pain (IASP), 1986)

This definition highlights that chronic or persistent pain can have different mechanisms. It may be caused by a disease such as arthritis which does not heal and causes ongoing damage. It may also be present in the absence of any tissue damage.

This is often difficult for healthcare professionals and patients to understand as generally pain indicates a response to a physical injury. However, there are situations when injury or damage has healed but the pain continues to be felt. This is due to an increase in the action potential output from the dorsal horn cells, leading to a condition known as 'wind-up' (Roberts, 2007).

CANCER PAIN

Cancer pain shares the same pathophysiological pathways as non-cancer pain. It can be a combination of nociceptive and neuropathic pain. Cancer pain can be due to direct invasion of the nerves by a tumour or by the compression of neighbouring tissues by the tumour which stimulates nociceptors. It can also be caused by treatments and procedures. Cancer pain has been described as a complicated persistent pain with many reasons causing that pain (Dickman, 2007). However, it is important to note that pain and cancer are not synonymous; a quarter of patients do not experience pain (Twycross et al., 2009).

CONCURRENT PAIN

Pain can be affected by many factors. Anxiety is known to heighten a patient's perception of pain; lack of sleep can decrease tolerance to pain. It is imperative that pain is assessed accurately and promptly so that appropriate interventions can be initiated. Interventions are beyond the limitations of this chapter and are, therefore, not going to be discussed. Pain is deemed such an important aspect of care that it has been suggested it be 'the fifth vital sign' (Joint Commission on Accreditation of Health Care Organisations, 2001). Pain can be an important sign to both the patient and the healthcare professional that there may be something wrong.

Unrelieved pain, particularly acute pain, can have both physiological and psychological negative outcomes. Some of the physiological complications have been identified by Chung and Lui (2003) who state that pain compromises the ability to cough or deep breathe, often resulting in atelectasis or pneumonia. Pain restricts mobility which may contribute to the development of deep vein thrombosis (DVT) and can interfere with sleep. Furthermore, pain intensifies stress hormone responses which can result in tissue breakdown, increased metabolic rate, blood clotting, water retention, and impaired immune function (Chung and Lui, 2003; Pritchard, 2009). Poorly managed pain can also lead to anxiety and altered pain perceptions (McMain, 2008). If pain is not treated effectively and left unaddressed, this can lead to central sensitisation and the possibility of patients going on to develop chronic pain conditions (Roberts, 2007). This can radically complicate a patient's recovery and lead to extended hospital stay and delays in discharge, with the resulting service and cost implications (MacLellan, 2004).

Pain can have a major effect on the sufferer's life. The odds of quitting one's job because of ill health are seven times higher among people experiencing chronic pain (Eriksen et al., 2003). With regard to chronic pain the Chief Medical Officer (2009) reported that chronic pain is more common now than it was 40 years ago and is having a significant effect on people's wellbeing, triggering sleeplessness, depression and impeding daily performance. It is a recurring source of disability with considerable psychological, social and economic consequences for the sufferer (Pain Coalition, 2007).

WHEN TO ASSESS PAIN?

Pain assessment should be a fundamental assessment undertaken on any admission to hospital, especially prior to and following surgery or following injury. Pain assessment should also be undertaken when patients are accepted to a new area for care, whether that is in hospital or the community setting. Furthermore, if there is a change in the patient's condition or if you suspect the patient has pain, assessment should be initiated. It is important to consider the best time to assess pain. When patients are at rest they are less likely to be experiencing pain. MacIntyre and Ready (2002) suggest that a better indicator of the effectiveness of analgesic interventions is an assessment of pain caused by physical activity such as coughing, deep breathing or movement. Regular assessment is imperative to ensure pain is managed effectively (Australian and New Zealand College of Anaesthetists, 2010).

All healthcare professionals have a responsibility to assess patients' pain. The Working Party Report by the Royal College of Surgeons and Royal College of Anaesthetists (1990) recommended the concept of specialist pain management services to help deal with managing patients' pain. However, pain assessment and management is an essential skill that all healthcare professionals should be versed in and it should not be left solely to the experts. It is an issue for all healthcare professionals in both primary and secondary care (Endacott et al., 2009).

GETTING READY TO PERFORM THE SKILL

EQUIPMENT

Pain may be assessed by the use of observation, questioning and assessment tools. The choice of tool will depend greatly on the patient who is to be assessed. The tool may consist of pictures, words or numbers. Alternatively it may consist of a series of questions or a set of observations the healthcare professional may need to undertake. Recognised pain assessment tools allow efficient communication and assessment by reducing the chance of error or bias. Written information increases compliance and helps patients feel in control and improves clinical outcomes. For patients unable to communicate their pain, either verbally or by using aids, behavioural or physiological assessments are particularly important (Davis, 2000). Remember, it is the quality of the assessment process that is important and not the tool being used.

CONSENT

It is essential that the consent of the patient is gained. This is to ensure that the patient (where able) can engage in the assessment and thus feel empowered.

COMMUNICATION SKILLS

Undertaking good pain assessment requires substantial communication with the patient. Listening to the patient helps to develop a therapeutic relationship which helps to reduce anxiety and pain levels (Walker et al., 2004). Assessing a patient requires time and good interviewing skills. For those patients not able to communicate fully or easily then observational skills are required.

PRIOR KNOWLEDGE

An understanding of the physiology of the nervous system, particularly how pain is transmitted, is beneficial. Also knowledge and understanding of the different types of pain that the patient may be experiencing would be advantageous.

PROCEDURE – UNDERTAKING AN INITIAL PAIN ASSESSMENT

It is important to undertake pain assessment using a systematic approach to ensure that all information is gathered and valuable information is not missed.

Table 5.1

Action	Rationale
Introduce yourself to the patient	To establish a rapport with the patient and to gain patient cooperation
Explain what you are going to do	Patients often do not feel empowered and are unsure of their role in their own pain management (MacLellan, 2004). By explaining the assessment process and the relevance of that assessment, patients may feel empowered in their own care
Gain consent to carry out the assessment	To ensure patient cooperation as self reports of pain are accepted as the gold standard
Questions to ask the patient	
• Where is the pain?	To identify the location and possible cause, also to eliminate any assumptions by the healthcare professional.
• Does the pain radiate to anywhere else?	To identify other areas affected and possible causes. For example, pain at the tip of the shoulder blade can indicate cholecystitis
• When did the pain start?	To identify if the pain is acute or chronic
• Have you experienced this pain before?	To recognise whether this is a new or previously known pain
• How severe is the pain? A pain assessment tool may assist with this aspect	To indicate the significance and urgency of the situation for the patient
• Can you describe the pain?	A description of the pain may help to identify the type of pain
• Is it there all the time or does it come and go?	To help identify the cause of the pain as some conditions may cause continuous pain, while with others the pain varies
• Does anything make it better?	To identify what strategies may improve the situation
• Does anything make it worse?	To identify any triggering factors, e.g. whether movement increases pain or it follows eating
• How does the pain affect your daily life activities?	To determine the effect of pain on the patient's physical, psychological and psycho-social wellbeing.
• Do you normally take any analgesic (pain killing) medication?	To ascertain the patient's current analgesic intake (if any)

(Continued)

Table 5.1   (Continued)

Action	Rationale
Document the results of the assessment	Following any assessment it is important to document all information. The assessment may need to be repeated if the patient reports changes to their pain. Further assessments may be recorded on the appropriate assessment tool or observation chart. Other colleagues or health professionals involved in the patient's care can use the results to evaluate interventions throughout the episode of care
Report any changes	To ensure appropriate action can be taken. A sudden change in pain experience could indicate the development of a new problem or deterioration in condition

POINTS TO NOTE

- **Age** – It is important to consider the age of the individual whom you are assessing. Different communication skills, observational skills and assessment tools may be required depending upon the age of the patient. For example, neonates, pre-verbal children, school children and elderly patients may all need an adaptation to the way in which assessment is undertaken.
- **Mental Capacity** – The ability of the patient to comprehend what you are trying to achieve is an important factor to consider. Individuals who have learning difficulties, cognitive impairment such as dementia or those with mental health problems will require careful attention to ensure an appropriate assessment is fulfilled.
- **Language** – This does not refer solely to the fact that patients we care for may speak a different language than we do but also that the words we choose may have different meanings to our patients. The meaning of words and colloquial use may also alter understanding. For example, the use of the term 'moderate pain' may not be understood by patients or have little relevance to their individual descriptions of pain (Mackintosh, 2005). For those patients who speak a language different to our own, an interpreter will be required.
- **Observation** – The emotional and physical indicators of pain are useful, whether the patient can communicate with the practitioner or not. Observing body language and facial expressions may contribute to the pain assessment. For example, as you approach a patient they may appear fidgety, changing position regularly, restless, holding or rubbing parts of their body. Facial expressions may be tense, frowning, grimacing or angry. These may all be an indication of pain and can be vital, particularly if the patient is unable or reluctant to report pain levels. For those patients who are unable to verbalise their pain, important additional information may be gained from family or carers.
- **Gender** – It is important to consider that men and women may react differently to pain and that this may impact on assessment.

- **Culture** – Diverse cultures may have different beliefs regarding pain and the expression of that pain.
- **Previous Experience** – Whether a person has had a positive or negative previous experience of pain can have an impact on how they react when faced with a painful situation in the future.
- **Meaning of Pain** – Pain can have different meanings for people throughout their lives. For example, for those suffering from cancer pain Cherny and Portenoy (2005: 787) suggest that 'In the cancer population, assessment must recognise the dynamic relationship between the symptom, the illness, and larger concerns related to quality of life'.
- **Health Professionals' Attitude** – Health professionals have their own views and preconceived ideas regarding pain. This can lead to patients' pain being underestimated (White, 2004). It is important that all staff who play a part in assessing patients' pain put aside their own feelings and concentrate on the patient.
- **Reassessment** – For pain to be managed successfully, pain must be assessed/reassessed regularly and appropriate action must be taken according to the outcome of that assessment.
- **Concurrent Pain** – Patients may experience more than one pain at a time. For example, a patient may have rheumatoid arthritis and be undergoing a surgical procedure which would cause acute pain.
- **Threshold and Tolerance** – Pain threshold refers to the level of stimulation at which pain is experienced. Tolerance refers to a person's ability to bear pain with regard to its intensity and duration. Tolerance can vary from person to person; it can also differ within the same person at different times.

CONCLUSION

The importance of pain assessment has been discussed and shown to be a significant skill to master. Knowledge of different types of pain and the other factors which may influence a patient's perception of pain are important issues to consider when undertaking pain assessment. It is a complex topic and the ability to undertake pain assessment effectively will ultimately improve the experience for your patient, will help to speed recovery and ultimately reduce the amount of unnecessary suffering.

Introduction

The following scenario is designed to assist healthcare professionals to undertake a comprehensive pain assessment. The scenario may be adapted as required to suit other healthcare settings. Specific pain assessment tools may be incorporated into the scenario as required.

Learning Objectives

By the end of this scenario the healthcare professional will be able to:

- Identify the equipment required to undertake a pain assessment
- Recognise the communication skills required to enable successful pain assessment
- Demonstrate the skill required to undertake pain assessment.

SIMULATION SCENARIO

Resources

- List of questions or appropriate pain assessment tool (see Table 5.1 for questions)
- Pen and paper to simulate documentation
- Three chairs for participants.

Setting

This scenario could be performed in a classroom setting, as a small group exercise, or incorporated into a clinical skill simulation.

Time element

- 20 minutes for assessment
- 10 minutes for discussion.

Scenario

Jack is a 74-year-old Caucasian gentleman who has undergone a replacement heart valve operation. He is generally fit and healthy with the only history to note being a traumatic amputation of his right arm from an industrial accident 36 years ago.

He has been transferred from the high dependency unit to the cardiac surgery ward recently. On return from theatre Jack had a continuous morphine infusion but now he is tolerating food and fluids he has been prescribed oral paracetamol and codeine. He appears comfortable but staff have noticed that he is reluctant to cough or move. Jack needs to have a full pain assessment undertaken to establish how care needs to proceed.

Roles of Participants

- Facilitator to undertake the role of Jack
- One student to undertake the role of the health professional
- One student to observe.

Areas for Discussion

- Did the range of questions provide a comprehensive pain assessment?
- Did Jack answer all the questions?
- Were there any other questions you would have liked to have asked?
- Was any clarification required from Jack or the assessor to elicit a comprehensive response, e.g. rephrasing or repetition of questions?
- Did the observer notice anything regarding body language?
- How was the assessment documented? Was this difficult or easy? If an assessment tool was used, did it allow for all information gathered to be documented?

Points for Consideration

A patient's age, cognitive ability, gender, culture and previous experiences may all influence how a patient perceives pain. Patients regularly come into our care and expect to experience pain from surgery or procedures. All too often this is exactly what they experience. With the skills to assess pain accurately patients will benefit and their experiences will greatly improve.

REFERENCES

Angell, M. (1982) 'The quality of mercy', *New England Journal of Medicine*, 306 (2): 98–9.

Australian and New Zealand College of Anaesthetists and Faculty of Pain Medicine (2010) *Acute Pain Management: Scientific Evidence*, 3rd edn. Melbourne: ANZCA and FPM.

Bell, L. and Duffy, A. (2009) 'Pain assessment in surgical nursing: a literature review', *British Journal of Nursing*, 18 (3): 151–6.

Burglass, L. (2007) 'The assessment of acute pain in adults', in K. McGann (ed.), *Fundamental Aspects of Pain Assessment and Management*. Tyne and Wear: Quay Books Division.

Cherny, N.I. and Portenoy, R.K. (2005) 'Cancer pain: principles of assessment and syndromes', in S. McMahon and M. Koltzenburg (eds) *Wall and Melzack's Textbook of Pain*. London: Elsevier, Chapter 43.

Chief Medical Officer (2010) *Annual Report*. London: DH.

Chung, J. and Lui, J. (2003) 'Postoperative pain management: study of patients' level of pain and satisfaction with healthcare providers' responsiveness to their reports of pain', *Nursing and Health Sciences*, 5: 13–21.

Davis, B. (2000) *Caring for People in Pain*. London: Routledge.

Dickman, A. (2007) 'Pain in palliative care: a review', *Pharmaceutical Journal*, 278: 679–82.

Dihle, A., Bjolseth, G. and Helseth, S. (2006) 'The gap between saying and doing in post operative pain management', *Journal of Clinical Nursing*, 15 (4): 469–79.

Endacott, R., Jevon, P. and Cooper, S. (2009) *Clinical Nursing Skills. Core and Advanced*. Oxford: Oxford University Press.

Eriksen, J., Jensen, M., Sjogren, P., Ekholm, O. and Rasmussen, N. (2003) 'Epidemiology of chronic non malignant pain in Denmark', *Pain*, 106 (3): 221–8.

Healthcare Commission (2006) *National Survey of Adult Inpatients*. Available on: http://www.nhssurveys.org/survey/561 [accessed 4 November 2011].

International Association for the Study of Pain (IASP) (1986) *Classification of Chronic Pain. Descriptions of Chronic Pain Syndromes and Definitions of Pain Terms*. Prepared by the ISAP Subcommittee on Taxonomy. Pain Suppl., S1–S226.

International Association for the Study of Pain (IASP) (2010) *Declaration of Montreal; Declaration that Access to Pain Management Is a Fundamental Human Right*. Available on http://www.iasppain.org/Content/NavigationMenu/Advocacy/DeclarationofMontr233al/default.htm [accessed 4 November 2011].

Joint Commission on Accreditation of Health Care Organisations (2001) *Pain: Current Understanding of Assessment Management and Treatments*. Oakbrook Terrace, IL: JCAH and the National Pharmaceutical Council, National Pharmaceutical Council, Inc.

MacIntyre, P. and Ready, L. (2002) *Acute Pain Management; A Practical Guide*, 2nd edn. Edinburgh: WB Saunders.

Mackintosh, C. (2005) 'Appraising pain', in C. Banks and K. Mackrodt (eds), *Chronic Pain Management*. London: Whurr Publishers. pp. 92–112.

MacLellan, K. (2004) 'Postoperative pain: strategy for improving patients' experiences. Issues and interventions in nursing practice', *Journal of Advanced Nursing*, 46 (2): 179–85.

McCaffery, M. (1979) *Nursing Management of the Patient with Pain*. Philadelphia, PA: Lippincott.

McMain, L. (2008) 'Principles of acute pain management', *Pain Management*, 18 (11): 473–8.

Merskey, H. and Bogduk, N. (1994) *Classification of Chronic Pain: Description of Chronic Pain Syndromes and Definitions of Pain Terms*, 2nd edn. Seattle, WA: IASP Press.

Pain Coalition (2007) http://www.paincoalition.org.uk/cppc [accessed 15 January 2011].

Pritchard, J. (2009) 'Managing anxiety in the elective surgical patient', *British Journal of Nursing*, 18 (7): 416–20.

Roberts, A. (2007) 'The management of acute pain', in K. McGann (ed.), *Fundamental Aspects of Pain Assessment and Management*. Tyne and Wear: Quay Books.

Royal College of Anaesthetists (2003) *Pain Management Services Good Practice*. London: RCA.

The Royal College of Surgeons and the Royal College of Anaesthetists (1990) *Commission on the Provision of Surgical Services. Report of the Working Party on Pain after Surgery*. London: RCS.

Sjöström, B., Dahlgren, L. and Haljamane, H. (2000) 'Strategies used in post operative pain assessment and their clinical accuracy', *Journal of Clinical Nursing*, 9 (1): 111–118.

Sloman, R., Rosen, G., Rom, M. and Shir, Y. (2005) 'Nurses' assessment of pain in surgical patients', *Journal of Advanced Nursing*, 52 (2): 125–32.

Twycross, R., Wilcock, A. and Stark Toller, C. (2009) *Symptom Management in Advanced Cancer*, 4th edn. Nottingham: Palliative Drugs.com.

Walker, J., Payne, S., Smith, P. and Jarrett, N. (2004) *Psychology for Nurses and the Caring Professions*. Berkshire: Open University Press.

White, S. (2004) 'Assessment of chronic neuropathic pain and the use of pain tools', *British Journal of Nursing*, 13 (7): 372–8.

6

ACTING IN EMERGENCIES: BLS AND SUMMONING ASSISTANCE

Paul Knott

Aim

This chapter describes the fundamental skills of effective basic life support (BLS) and includes a practical step-by-step approach to running a basic life support simulation and basic skills assessment toolkit.

Objectives

To understand and discuss:

- The importance of summoning prompt assistance in an emergency situation
- The identification of the key issues, correct sequence and technique for performing effective basic life support
- The use of SBAR as a communication tool in critical situations.

INTRODUCTION TO THE SKILL

Basic life support is often described as the 'cornerstone of resuscitation' and is an essential part of the chain of survival, as described by the Resuscitation Council UK (2010).

The brain appears to accumulate ischemic injury faster than any other organ. Full recovery of the brain after more than three minutes of cardiac arrest at normal body temperature without treatment is rare (Safar, 1986, 1988).

Basic life support (BLS), also often referred to interchangeably as cardiopulmonary resuscitation or CPR, is an amalgamation of looking for signs of life in the collapsed patient, opening the airway, and providing chest compressions and artificial ventilation. It is emphasised (Resuscitation Council UK, 2010) that BLS is a holding measure that will maintain viability in terms of cell survival until the availability of means of restarting the heart of a victim of cardiac arrest. A simple mnemonic (the DRS' ABC) may be used in order to remind of the correct sequencing:

'DRS ABC':
D – Danger
R – Response
S – Shout for help
A – Airway
B – Breathing
C – Circulation/compressions

Effective training is an essential ingredient in the development of competence for the healthcare professional. Eder-Van Hook (2004: 2) states that 'A healthcare provider's ability to react prudently in an unexpected situation is one of the most critical factors in creating a positive outcome in medical emergency'. According to Nishisaki et al. (2007), simulation training improves provider and team self-efficacy and competence on manikins, and there is some evidence to suggest procedural simulation improves actual operational performance in clinical settings.

The use of patient simulation manikins enables the learner to bridge the theory–practice gap by acting out realistic simulations of real life events, without putting patients at risk. Scenarios can be repeated with consistency and this provides a benchmark to assess levels of competence and provide evidence for continuing professional development. The author suggests that with the development of high cost, high fidelity manikins, healthcare professionals may be overwhelmed by equipment fidelity and focus on this rather than the planned teaching and learning that is taking place. Some studies, such as Bell et al. (2008), demonstrated no significant difference in second year doctors' resuscitation performance skills when comparing two groups who had received high and low fidelity training.

GETTING READY TO PERFORM THE SKILL

The rescuer should consider scene safety and immediate risk assessment to be of paramount importance. Dependent on the environment, the rescuer should look for such dangers as listed in Table 6.1.

Table 6.1

External environment	Clinical area
Traffic if in a street environment	Furniture/equipment around the patient's bedside
Falling debris from overhead	Bodily fluids
Fire/chemicals	Used needles or other sharps
Electricity/water	Trailing cables from monitors

PERFORMING BASIC LIFE SUPPORT

Table 6.2

Action	Rationale
• **D**anger • Risks to the rescuer	Assess the area for risks and make a careful approach to the patient looking for dangers, as per Table 6.1
• Check the patient for a **R**esponse by gently shaking the patient's shoulders, while holding the head still, verbalising 'Are you OK?'	Is the patient just asleep or truly unconscious? Stabilise the head in case a cervical spine injury is present. Shake the shoulders in case the patient is hearing impaired or semi-conscious
• **S**hout for help	Ensure your colleagues or bystanders are aware you have an emergency situation and activate the emergency bell system if available. If no one responds to your call for help then you must call for emergency assistance before commencing CPR. As students might be keen to get on with CRR, it may be helpful to state why you will require help at some point (single responder CPR not possible for prolonged period)
• Open the **A**irway using the head tilt chin lift (see Figure 6.1), consider jaw thrust only if cervical spine injury, and check for **B**reathing and for signs of life (**C**irculation) using the Look, Listen and Feel approach	Consider simultaneously maintaining a head tilt chin lift and carotid pulse check Look for chest rise, listen for air entry and exit at the mouth and feel for air movement against your cheek This rapid clinical assessment should be completed in less than 10 seconds

(Continued)

Table 6.2   (Continued)

Action	Rationale
• If a pulse is palpable or signs of life are present, urgent medical assessment is required. Maintain the patient's airway using the head tilt chin lift position and reassess using the ABCDE approach	Maintaining the patient's airway is of crucial importance. The patient must be monitored continually for signs of deterioration as they are at high risk of further deterioration into cardio-respiratory arrest and, if this occurs, CPR should be commenced immediately
• If the patient is not breathing but has a palpable pulse then this is considered to be a respiratory arrest and rescue breaths should be commenced at the rate of 10–12 breaths per minute	A patient may be in respiratory arrest alone and rescue breathing should be commenced to support the patient. A full pulse check should only be performed if the practitioner is experienced and confident in doing so. If pulse is unable to be checked, then the absence of breathing in an adult victim is enough to commence full CPR (Resuscitation Council UK, 2010)
• If available, send an assistant to call for assistance and gain early access to advanced life support personnel. In the UK the national emergency number within an NHS hospital with a cardiac arrest team is 2222 (National Patient Safety Agency, 2004). • In clinical circumstances and in the community where a local cardiac arrest team is not accessible an emergency ambulance must be called without delay	Summoning help and early defibrillation is of paramount importance. For the patient that presents in a shockable rhythm for every minute's delay in access to and use of a defibrillator there is a 10–15% loss of survival (Resuscitation Council UK, 2010). Many public locations now have access to Automated External Defibrillators (AED) and this should be asked for when requesting help
• For the patient who shows no signs of life, commence chest compressions with your palms in the middle of the lower part of the sternum NOTE: Occasional gasps may be an indication of agonal breathing and is not a sign of life. If agonal breathing is suspected CPR should commence immediately	The performance of high quality chest compressions is of paramount importance to improve survival. The Resuscitation Council UK (2010) cites the following parameters for effective chest compressions: ○ Depth of 5–6 cm ○ Rate of 100–120 chest compressions per minute ○ Allow the chest to recoil completely after each chest compression Timing devices built into the AED to coach the rescuer into performing high quality chest compressions are

(Continued)

Table 6.2   (Continued)

Action	Rationale
	becoming more commonplace as technology evolves and improves. These devices now enable the lay rescuer with limited or even no training the opportunity to perform defibrillation for the first time. They may also provide a coaching facility to assist in improving the quality of CPR by providing a simple metronome 'bleep', voice commands such as 'press one, press two, press three' or incorporate sophisticated feedback sensors which monitor chest compressions and give feedback to the rescuer such as 'press a little faster'
• Provide a ratio of 30 chest compressions followed by two ventilations	Mouth-to-mouth resuscitation may not be aesthetically appealing to the rescuer, especially if the victim is unknown to them. In the absence of barrier devices such as a pocket mask or bag valve mask, consider chest compression only CPR until this facility becomes available
• Use of mouth-to-pocket mask ventilation	Mouth-to-pocket masks to provide positive pressure ventilation from exhaled breath have several advantages. They are small and therefore portable. They are relatively cheap and therefore commonly available. Pocket masks may also provide the rescuer with some level of protection regarding cross infection as it contains a physical barrier by means of the mask and one-way valve (Resuscitation Council UK, 2010). If oxygen is available, the rescuer's exhaled breath can be enriched to provide a higher concentration of oxygen by attaching the pocket mask to a built-in side port or by simply putting the open end of oxygen tubing between the patient's face and the mask. Oxygen flows should be the maximum available
• Use of bag valve mask ventilation	When used with high flow oxygen (15 litres) and a reservoir attachment, a bag valve mask will achieve up to 90% oxygen delivery

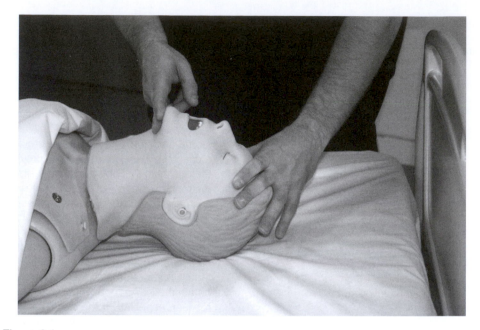

Figure 6.1

COMMUNICATION STRATEGIES IN EMERGENCY SITUATIONS

Emergency situations can occur infrequently; skills rehearsal and simulation activity provides learners with the opportunity to practise in a safe environment with the ultimate aim of bridging the theory–practice gap.

Communication is often problematic in unplanned emergency situations where members of the multidisciplinary healthcare professional team, who may not know one another, are expected to deal with an emergency in stressful situations. The use of structured communication tools are becoming more commonplace in an effort to address this and provide the learner with a useful guide to practise clear communication in role-play scenario sessions. Evidence is available that suggests that the use of structured communication tools improves interdisciplinary communication (Marshall et al., 2009). A commonly cited example of this type of tool is 'Situation, Background, Assessment, Recommendation (SBAR)' (National Health Improvement Agency, 2008). An example dialogue is illustrated in Table 6.3.

CONCLUSION

Due to better early recognition of the deteriorating patient, cardiac arrests are becoming less frequent within the clinical environment. However, basic life support

Table 6.3

Situation	Introduce self and whom the focus of the discussion is about Use patient identifiers to reduce the risk of error Identify the problem or perceived problem For example: 'I need some advice on ...' 'The problem appears to be ...'
Background	About the patient 'This 55-year-old patient came in by ambulance 15 minutes ago and has chest pains'
Assessment	Provide a list of current vital signs 'He appears to be deteriorating and his Early Warning Score is ... '
Recommendation	State what you require of the person 'I think you should come and see him right away please' 'Is there anything you would like me to do in the meantime?'

Source: Adapted from National Health Improvement Agency, 2008

(BLS) is a skill which all healthcare practitioners should be competent in providing. The use of simulated training in this area can help to promote a deeper understanding and prepare the practitioner for dealing with an emergency in a systematic and timely manner. This should, in turn, help to provide a better patient outcome in this situation. Communication when dealing with an emergency is of paramount importance and must be highlighted to the learners throughout their training. The use of a shared mental model such as 'SBAR' can help to facilitate effective communication and summon assistance among healthcare professionals.

Environment

Consider the location of the session carefully. A simple way of achieving realism is to run training within the learners' clinical area. The surroundings, emergency equipment and facilities such as emergency call buzzers will be familiar to the learners and this provides a low-cost option as these facilities are already there. However, it is clearly not always practical to use the clinical environment, especially if patients are present, in which case a suitable training area should be selected that can be arranged in a way that represents the students' workplace.

Ground Rules

In clinical skills the physical activity of performing skills can be embarrassing for the learner. This is particularly so if they have not had exposure to this type of training before, that is, training which includes the concepts of role-play and patient simulators. Safety is considered one of the basic human requirements within Maslow's hierarchy of needs (Maslow, 1954) and it is unlikely that learners will reach their full potential within a session if they do not feel safe. It is important, therefore, to discuss

SIMULATION SCENARIO

and agree ground rules regarding mutual expectations and set an environment in which the learners feel comfortable.

It is helpful to rationalise the skills-teaching activity as an opportunity to practise, make errors and improve clinical skills within a safe environment. If things don't go to plan, they can always be repeated – which is the clear benefit over real life.

Equipment Required for Running the Scenario

Table 6.4

Equipment required	Instructor notes
• Basic life support manikin	Consider the fidelity of available equipment. What do you intend to do? Consider a basic or more advanced manikin based on the intended scenario. Another consideration is the number of instructors you have available. Some high fidelity manikins require several operators to run a realistic scenario
• Consider use of the emergency trolley if used in clinical area	Ensure that you have spare equipment to replace what you have used
• Height adjustable bed or patient trolley	CPR is a physical skill and is also hard work! To achieve and demonstrate competence, learners will have to perform multiple chest compressions. To reduce the risk of injury to joints and especially the lower back, instruct learners to swap regularly during your scenarios. As an instructor you are ultimately responsible for the health and safety of your learners. Consider the build and height of your learners as an ongoing risk assessment. You may need to lower and heighten the bed between learners while in a teaching scenario
• Disposable gloves and defibrillator safety point	Standard barrier precautions should be emphasised during the session and this should include the use of gloves. Modern resuscitation and defibrillation techniques emphasise the need to reduce 'hands off time' where a team member continues chest compressions, colleagues stand clear and a defibrillator is simultaneously charged (See Figure 6.2) The team member providing the chest compressions moves away safely before the defibrillatory shock is administered. Not only do the gloves provide the learner with some degree of bacterial barrier but it has been suggested that they may provide the person undertaking chest compressions with insulation against the defibrillatory shock (Lloyd et al., 2008) should the defibrillator be accidentally discharged before they have stood clear

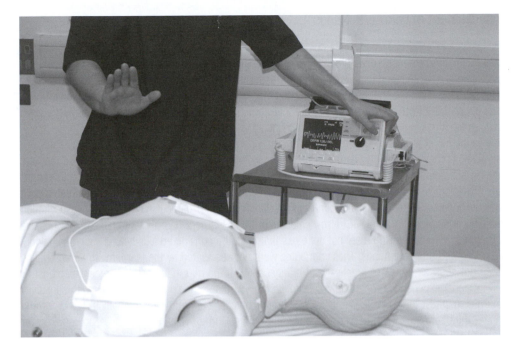

Figure 6.2

Table 6.5

Equipment required	Instructor notes
• Decontamination wipes and disposable manikin consumables	Check with the manikin manufacturer or representative for suitable disinfection products. Note: the specification of the manikin should be checked before running the scenario. Many modern manikins have relatively cheap consumable parts, such as replacement lungs and face skins, which should be replaced frequently as recommended by the manufacturer. It is important to note that just because a manikin has 'lungs' and is designed to illustrate ventilation does not necessarily mean that is it suitable for mouth-to-mouth. More advanced manikins may be designed for the exclusive use of bag valve mask ventilation and may or may not have the facility to receive more advanced airway adjuncts. The use of mouth-to-mouth or mouth-to-pocket mask may pose an infection control hazard to persons using the manikins if they are not designed for this purpose

Assessment of Learners' Needs

Resuscitation training is now fairly commonplace, with organisations such as the Red Cross and Saint John's Ambulance Service running regular training for the lay public in the UK. Many healthcare professionals are required to undertake regular resuscitation training and may have previous training or real-life experiences. It should be acknowledged that cardiopulmonary resuscitation can be an emotive subject and the instructor should be aware that demonstration of these skills can reveal unexpected hidden emotions in the learner and that these should be addressed sensitively.

Manderino et al. (1986) look at the physiological changes in learners performing within a healthcare simulation. They were able to demonstrate increases in pulse rate and blood pressure of the learners during a simulation of a cardiac arrest. It was suggested in the study that emotional thoughts trigger the physiological responses which were recorded in the study. The effect of physiological stress should not be underestimated within the simulation environment, with particular reference to resuscitation training. Manderino et al. (1986) also demonstrated that learners had an awareness of the positive attributes of an 'adrenaline rush' but not those that could be considered less helpful such as shaking, fumbling and dropping things. These attributes were not associated by the learner with an adrenaline rush but seen as a lack of practical and manual skills. If learners have had any recent personal or professional experiences regarding resuscitation the instructor should deal with these with sensitivity as they manifest themselves. The instructor should consider the organisation in which they work and make themselves aware of any relevant student counselling services should these be required for referral following the session.

The four-stage approach, as described by Bullock et al. (2008), is commonly used in resuscitation skills training and is used here to develop the learner's ability to apply the skills observed to their own patient simulation experience. The four-stage approach is summarised in the Table 6.6.

Table 6.6

Stage 1
Put the skill into context by providing a demonstration with limited or no dialogue

Stage 2
Perform the skill again with full description, allowing learners the opportunity to ask questions

Stage 3
Perform the skill again while guided by the learners. If there is a particularly strong learner, select them. Alternatively, consider asking several learners. It is important that you correct any errors and again clarify any questions. Questions in both directions help to clarify the learning

Stage 4
Invite a learner to perform the skill. The learner group can support him/her. This provides a valuable peer learning opportunity as learners naturally fill in each other's knowledge gaps. It also makes the learner performing the skill feel less anxious about performing the skill for the first time in front of the peer group and completes any knowledge gaps

---

Stage 1

Table 6.7

Content	Demonstration
• Set the scene and context of the simulation so that it makes sense to the learner within your chosen teaching environment. Where are you? What are you doing? What is your role? • Perform the skill in real time with limited verbal dialogue so the simulation is understood by the learner. This is your opportunity to act as a role model. The skills performed must be accurate	Perform the skill around a basic scenario that meets the learner's needs and assessment criteria

Stage 2

Table 6.8

Content	Demonstration
• Repeat the skill	Repeat the skill and demonstration as set out in Stage 1 but at a slower pace with commentary. It is important that the learners have the opportunity to ask questions
• Consider the room layout; can your learners see?	This is an appropriate time to invite learners up to see more clearly as you demonstrate the skills. Airway skills in particular can be difficult to see; learners should be invited to stand, move closer and orientate their view to ensure understanding

Instructor Notes

Consider the use of own clinical practice and experiences of the group to underpin the techniques. Allow the flow of natural discussion and deal with questions as they arise. Avoid 'shelving' a question until later if it can be addressed at the time.

Stage 3

In this stage there is a shift from the didactic approach as responsibility for the skill moves from instructor to learner.

Table 6.9

Content	Demonstration
• Repeat the simulation scenario guided by one of the learners	In a weaker learner group, consider having the whole group guide this activity. This is a particularly valuable stage in the learning process; peer-to-peer learning takes place and it gives the instructor the opportunity to make a judgement on the learners' learning at this point. It allows the opportunity to alter the pace, content and explanation of the skill to suit the learners' needs

Stage 4

Allow learners the opportunity to practise the same scenario with instructor correction as required. Facilitate the smooth running of the scenario with peer feedback to guide the learner performing the skill. To ensure that the learner feels supported and to limit any performance anxiety in front of the peer group, remind the learner that this is the first practice experience and that the group will help them if required.

The instructor should continually assess the level of knowledge, competence, engagement and enthusiasm of the learners during this stage and when selecting further learners to perform the skills for themselves. An awareness of learning preferences should also be considered. Some learners may wish to have a go to 'get it over with' while others will prefer to watch and reflect on what they have seen of their peers' performance before attempting their own scenario.

Points to Note

The depth and rate of chest compressions can be difficult to achieve consistently. It is important that the instructor demonstrates a consistent rate of 100–120 chest compressions per minute. This can be achieved through practice using a simple timing device such as a second hand on a watch (up to but not more than two chest compressions per second), metronome, mobile phone applications that provide a consistent audible beep. As technology continually improves, there are now timing devices built in to defibrillators that monitor the depth, rate and pauses (hands-off time) in chest compressions. If this is available in the learners' clinical area, these devices help to reduce the subjectivity in teaching and assessing the performance of these skills. In clinical practice team members may feel uncomfortable providing real-time feedback on the chest compression performances of others, especially as cardiac arrests are usually unexpected events and highly stressful for team members. An automated device may be advantageous by giving feedback in these circumstances.

Assessment Criteria

The role of the learner will dictate the learning outcomes within the session. Consider the following lists in Tables 6.10 and 6.11 as a basis for basic observational assessment.

Table 6.10

Observation Criteria	Evidence
• Safe approach	Observe the learner approach with care. If something naturally 'gets in the way', such as ECG leads or defibrillator pad leads, this can be a discussion point at the end of the simulation
• Assess for response	Observe the learner's approach to the patient and assessment of the patient for unconsciousness by shaking the shoulders and speaking as appropriate
• Open airway • Checks for ABC and/ or signs of life	(i) Observe a head tilt chin lift with a signs of life check (ii) Alternatively, a head tilt chin lift, carotid pulse check *and* signs of life check

Table 6.11

Observation Criteria	Evidence
• Calls for cardiac arrest team or ambulance depending on clinical setting	This is an important step in clear communication. Consider the level of fidelity and realism of the session. Do you have use of a phone? If possible have another facilitator answer the phone and play the role of the operator
• Commences chest compressions: (i) Hand position (ii) Body position (iii) Depth (iv) Recoil (v) Rate	Minimises rescuer fatigue through teamwork to maintain continuous chest compressions Consider how you are going to measure criteria (i)–(v) Are you going to use a stop watch? Are there adjuncts built into the equipment in the learner's clinical area? Many manikins record this information and can generate reports
• Effective use of pocket mask and/or • Effective use of bag valve mask	Observe a good seal and that the chest rises and falls Head tilt, chin lift Learner should request high flow oxygen Ventilating issues are a common problem in manikins. Ensure your equipment is working and 'plumbed in'. Many ventilation issues can be easily fixed by reconnecting a plastic tube within the manikin's chest. Check manufacturer's troubleshooting guidance or local technician

REFERENCES

Bell, G., Weidman, E.K., Walsh, D., Small, S., Abella, B.S., Vanden Hoek, T., Becker, L.B. and Edelson, D.P. (2008) *A Randomized Study of High-Fidelity Simulation Training on Actual Cardiopulmonary Resuscitation Performance.* Circulation 118:S_766, American Heart Association. Hagerstown: Lippincott Williams & Wilkins.

Bullock, I., Davis, M., Lockey, A. and Mackway-Jones, K. (2008) *Pocket Guide to Teaching for Medical Instructors,* 2nd edn. Oxford: Blackwell Publishing. pp. 39–41.

Eder-Van Hook, J. (2004) *Building a National Agenda for Simulation-based Medical Education.* Washington, DC: Telemedicine and Advanced Technology Research Centre (TATRC). p. 2.

Lloyd, M.S., Heeke, B., Walter, P.F. and Langberg, J.J. (2008) 'Hands-on defibrillation: an analysis of electrical current flow through rescuers in direct contact with patients during biphasic external defibrillation', *Circulation,* 117: 2510–14.

Manderino, M., Yonkman, C., Ganong, L. and Royal, A. (1986) 'Evaluation of a cardiac arrest simulation', *Journal of Nursing Education,* 25: 3: 107–11.

Marshall, S., Harrison, J. and Flanagan, B. (2009) 'The teaching of a structured tool improves the clarity and content of interprofessional clinical communication', *Qual Saf Health Care,* 18: 137–40.

Maslow, A. (1954) *Motivation and Personality.* New York: Harper and Row. p. 91.

National Health Improvement Agency (NHS) (2008*) Quality and Service Improvement Tools.* Available on: http://www.institute.nhs.uk/quality_and_service_improvement_tools/ quality_and_service_improvement_tools/sbar_-_situation_-_background_-_assessment_-_ recommendation.html [accessed 1 February 2011].

National Patient Safety Agency (2004) *Establishing a Standard Crash Call Telephone Number in Hospitals.* Patient safety alert 02. London: NPSA (NHS).

Nishisaki, A., Keren, R. and Nadkarni, V. (2007) 'Does simulation improve patient safety? Self-efficacy, competence, operational performance, and patient safety', *Anesthesiol Clin,* 25 (2): 225–36.

Resuscitation Council UK (2010) *Advanced Life Support,* 6th edn. London: Resuscitation Council.

Safar, P. (1986) 'Cerebral resuscitation after cardiac arrest, a review', *Circulation,* 74 (Suppl IV): 138–53.

Safar, P. (1988) 'Resuscitation from clinical death: pathophysiologic limits and therapeutic potentials', *Critical Care Medicine,* 16 (10): 923–41.

7

PERSONAL HYGIENE: BED BATH AND ORAL CARE

Barry Ricketts

Aim

The aim of this chapter is to support the practitioner to develop the required skills, knowledge and attitude relating to the principles of personal hygiene care in health and social care settings. This may relate to primary, secondary and tertiary settings where a client receives care; for example, a client's home, a consulting room, a hospital setting or any treatment and clinical area.

Objectives

The objectives are to:

- Discuss the factors to consider when assessing the client's needs for personal hygiene
- To identify ways to maintain a client's dignity and privacy when providing personal hygiene care
- Demonstrate how to provide personal care to a client, including bathing, skin care, mouth care and eye care.

INTRODUCTION TO THE SKILL AND EXPLANATION OF ITS IMPORTANCE

This skills section focuses on providing comfort and hygiene. It will cover the principles of providing personal care, including bathing, skin care, mouth care and eye care, while maintaining a client's privacy and dignity.

Personal hygiene care is:

> the physical act of cleansing the body to ensure that the hair, nails, ears, eyes, nose and skin are maintained in an optimum condition. It also includes mouth hygiene which is the effective removal of plaque and debris to ensure the structures and tissues of the mouth are kept in a healthy condition. In addition, personal hygiene includes ensuring the appropriate length of nails and hair. (Department of Health (DH), 2010)

The following key areas of healthcare practice will also be considered during this chapter in relation to personal hygiene, bed bathing and oral care:

- Risk assessment
- Assessment of the client's needs
- Communication skills
- Providing comfort
- Standard precautions
- Therapeutic relationships
- Understanding and interpreting non-verbal behaviour
- Moving and handling principles
- Use of research and evidence-based practice.

BACKGROUND TO THE SKILL

The aim of this tool is to help practitioners to take a client-focused (DH, 2010) and structured approach in order to offer good quality care and best practice in relation to personal hygiene. During the session practitioners will have the opportunity to demonstrate as well as discuss these skills with their peers and facilitators.

Personal hygiene and oral healthcare is an essential component of daily hygiene for hospitalised patients and for those patients cared for in the community. The ability to maintain personal hygiene and oral healthcare is a fundamental role of the practitioner. People's personal hygiene needs and preferences should be met by the practitioner according to the client's individual and clinical needs (DH, 2010).

GETTING READY TO PERFORM THE SKILL

Personal hygiene: bed bath and oral care links to the following scientific knowledge; and an understanding of the following principles will assist the practitioner to implement effective assessment and evaluation of the care provided:

- Protection and Immunity – infection, allergies, anaphylaxis, vaccinations, antibodies, antigens, antibiotics, autoimmunity, innate immunity, skin as a barrier
- Senses – sensory receptors, special senses (vision, hearing, taste, smell, balance) somatic senses (touch, temperature, pain, itch, proprioception)
- Digestive System – oral cavity and dentition, taste, digestion and absorption
- Skeletal and Muscular Systems – articulations (fibrous, cartilaginous and synovial joints), bone growth and repair, types of muscles, muscle movement and development.

The practitioner will require relevant up-to-date theoretical knowledge, the ability to perform the skill safely and the ability to demonstrate an appropriate professional attitude.

PROCEDURE

Table 7.1

Action	Rationale
Informed consent to perform all aspects of personal hygiene: bed bath and oral care	*Provides individualised care maintaining the best interests of the client's needs at all times*
Introduce yourself, ask what the client would like to be called	Behaviour is in a professional manner and respects the client as an individual
Use open-ended questions Offer client opportunity to ask questions Check the client understands, offer explanations and answer any queries	Gains informed consent to carry out personal hygiene care. Care is given in a safe environment that is appropriate for the client, respecting his/her wishes at all times
Considers client's requests and adopts a non-discriminatory approach to care	Provides individualised care respecting client's privacy and dignity at all times and during each stage of the procedure

(Continued)

Table 7.1 (Continued)

Action	Rationale
Assesses the client's history and relevant medical condition	To consider what special attention may be required, e.g. pain, wounds, skin integrity, drains and infusions, client's mobility and cognitive function. The client's care is planned and continuously evaluated to meet needs and preferences
Collect all relevant equipment before commencing procedure	Clients have their toiletries to meet their needs and preferences. To minimise disruption once the procedure has started and to reduce exposure time

Bed Bath

Action	Rationale
Consider standard precautions and the use of personal protective equipment (PPE) before commencing the procedure, e.g. aprons and gloves	To avoid contamination of micro-organisms being transmitted from high risk body areas, e.g. genitals, groin and axillae
Prepare the environment so that surfaces are clear from clutter and are clean	Minimise obstacles and allow for easy access to equipment in a clean environment to reduce contamination
Close doors, curtains and windows, and minimise distraction and disturbance	Maintain privacy, dignity and respect of the client at all times
Carefully remove bed linen, disposing of it in the linen skip. Leave the client covered with a blanket	Reduce the risk of micro-organisms being in contact with skin and clothing. Reduce the risk of clothing and bedding becoming wet or soiled during the procedure
Change water frequently during the bathing of each skin region and ensure that it remains at the correct temperature for the client	Reduce risk of cross-contamination, maintain stable body temperature and patient comfort
Use separate flannels and disposable wipes for the face, the upper, the lower body and the genitalia	Soiled linen and wipes can be easily disposed of to minimise transmission and reduce the risk of cross-contamination
One practitioner to complete washing and one to complete drying – interchange roles as necessary. Wash skin areas furthest from the practitioner to avoid wetting dry areas and to address safe principles of moving and handling	Minimise exposure time and skin cooling period, promote independence as necessary and allow for patient preference

Action	Rationale
After seeking client's preference regarding skin cleanliness regime, assist as necessary to wash and dry the client's face, making sure to rinse thoroughly, avoiding the eyes	Prevent sore skin or contact with eyes
Assess the eye for any additional cleansing needs and assist the client if required	To prevent damage and treat infection or detect early signs of disease. Promote client to meet their own eye care needs
If any contaminations from the eye need to be removed, sterile 0.9% sodium chloride or sterile water can be used. Swab the unaffected eye first and bath the lids with the eyes closed using a lint-free swab. Clean the lower eye lid from the nasal corner outwards and repeat on the upper lid with the client looking down	Reduce risk of further injury, abrasion and cross-contamination
Keep exposure of the body to a minimum throughout the procedure	Maintain client privacy and dignity, maintain adequate skin and body temperature
Wash upper body area, to include back, arms, hands, torso and axillae checking for skin integrity in skin folds. For female patients particular attention should be given to under the breasts	Promote patient wellbeing and reduce risk of cross-contamination while assessing all skin areas for skin integrity, soreness and nail condition
Wash lower body area, to include legs and feet, drying methodically between toes whilst assessing if further podiatry intervention maybe required	Promote client wellbeing and reduce risk of cross-contamination and infection whilst assessing skin integrity and nail condition
Wash around the genitalia and sacral area, checking with the client if they would prefer to carry out their own personal care. Points to note: For female clients, wash from front to back. For male patients, draw back the foreskin when washing the penis	Promote client wellbeing and reduce risk of cross-contamination and infection whilst assessing skin integrity
Client assisted with personal clothing as soon as is appropriate	To maintain privacy and dignity
Client assisted as necessary to care for hair	To meet personal needs, respecting preferences and client's dignity
Client assisted with facial shaving and cosmetic application as necessary	To meet personal needs, respecting preferences and client's dignity

(Continued)

Table 7.1 (Continued)

Action	Rationale
Oral Care	
Assess client's preference for oral care and comfort	To meet personal needs, respecting preferences and client's dignity
Brush all tooth surfaces for at least 90 seconds twice daily using a soft toothbrush and toothpaste (see Figure 7.1)	To loosen debris and prevent dental caries
Floss at least once daily or as advised by clinician	To loosen debris and prevent dental caries
Offer bland mouth rinse twice daily – one tablespoon and swish in the oral cavity for 90 seconds	Bland rinses such as 0.9 % saline or sodium bicarbonate are used to remove loose debris and can aid with oral hydration.
Undertake an oral assessment to include tongue, lips and gums observing for redness, ulceration or bleeding	To monitor treatment to ensure a healthy mouth
Use water-based moisturisers to protect lips	To reduce incidence of cracking or ulceration and promotion of healthy lips

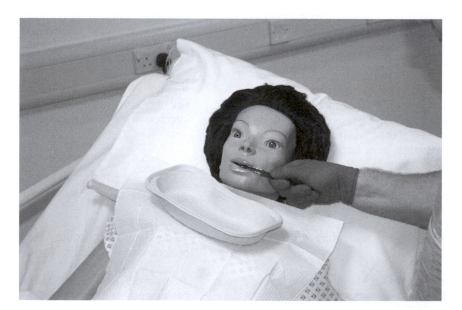

Figure 7.1

CONCLUSION – POINTS TO NOTE WHEN TEACHING AND PERFORMING THE SKILL

Consideration should be given to the following points:

- Independence – encourage independence at all times, by respecting the client's wishes
- Consent – ensure consent is sought before providing any treatment or intervention
- Personal preference – consider the client's personal preferences alongside any religious or cultural needs
- Privacy and dignity – maintain patient privacy as much as is possible and recognise that this may be harder to achieve in a hospital setting
- Warmth – clients may easily feel the cold, depending on the nature of the bed bath
- Water temperature – client preference can vary and, therefore, the temperature should be regulated accordingly throughout the procedure
- Comfort – client's position and bed bath comfort level should be confirmed throughout the procedure; this may vary if the client is bed bound, older or post-operative
- Risk assessment – consideration should be given to both the client and the practitioner. This may include moving and handling issues, standard precautions that must be instigated, pressure area risk assessment and contraindications for therapy
- Cleanliness and dryness of the skin – the client's preference may determine how hard the skin is dried and what agents are used. Consider allergies with respect to all products and therapies.

Bed Bath and Oral Care

Introduction to Simulation/Scenario

This skills session focuses on providing comfort and hygiene. It will cover the principles of providing personal care, including bathing, skin care, mouth care and eye care, while maintaining the client's privacy and dignity.

Practitioners are asked to bring in the following equipment: a selection of toiletries to use during the session including soap, flannel, towel, toothbrush and toothpaste, and to wear shorts and vest tops.

Learning Objectives

At the end of the simulation the student will be able to:

- Discuss the factors to consider when assessing the client's needs for personal hygiene care
- Identify ways to maintain a client's dignity when providing personal hygiene care
- Demonstrate how to provide personal care to a client, including bathing, care of skin, mouth care and eye care
- Assess clients through communication and interpretation of non-verbal behaviour, while providing comfort and hygiene care and while maintaining privacy and dignity
- Use research and evidence-based practice to inform principles of care.

SIMULATION SCENARIO

Resources Required for the Scenario

Equipment

- Manikins that can be washed and/or practitioners may act as a patient if undertaking experiential learning
- Clean night clothes
- Gloves, aprons, yellow clinical waste bags
- Clean linen and laundry skip, pillows, blankets, towels, flannels and, preferably, disposable wash cloths
- Wash bowls, soap, toothbrushes, toothpaste, eye care packs, saline and shaving items
- Mouth care packs, foam sticks, mouth care tablets, plastic cups, vomit bowls or kidney dishes
- Brush or comb, shampoo and conditioner
- Practitioners are asked to bring in the following equipment: a selection of toiletries to use during the session including: soap, flannel, towel, toothbrush and toothpaste, and to wear shorts and vest tops.

Setting

A clinical skills suite – that is, a simulated ward environment with beds containing curtains and bedside tables, with access to running water and appropriate clinical waste disposal is required.

Remember that the scenario could also be simulated within a client's home, clinic or hospital setting.

Time – Length of Session

Four hours is advised, however, this can be reviewed depending on how much practice is given to undertaking full hygiene care.

Situation/Scenario

The scenario can be tailored to meet the needs of the practitioner; this may include an acute care setting postoperative procedure, long-term community care or in the client's home. The dependence and acuity of the client can be determined by the prior experience of the practitioners and the specific predetermined learning outcomes.

Introduction to the Session

This includes the roles of participants with an explanation of their tasks (see Table 7.2).

Activity One: Individual Assessment of a Client's Personal Hygiene Needs (30 minutes)

The first activity is designed to help practitioners to think about the importance of an individual assessment of the client's hygiene needs. It also helps practitioners to consider some of the questions that they may need to ask the client, to seek further information about their hygiene needs.

1 Divide the practitioners into groups of three or complete this as one large group, depending on the number of practitioners. Ask the practitioners to discuss with each other one thing that is important to them in relation to their own hygiene needs, e.g. something you would not be able to go out of the house without doing. These may include washing hair daily, cleaning teeth before breakfast, a daily shower, a nightly bath, use of specific toiletries. Discuss how the group members all have different answers and regimes. This activity can identify the diversity and personal preferences among the group. Ask the practitioners to relate this to their individual assessment of a client's hygiene needs and what type of questions might now be relevant.

2 Ask the practitioners to share their answers to the following questions:

- When assessing a client's individual hygiene needs what factors do you think you would need to consider? (The facilitator may need to be available for guidance depending on the group's experience)
- Answers may include: level of ability to carry out own care, both cognitive ability and physical ability; mobility and restrictions due to situation, e.g. lines, drains, health status, pain; personal preferences, e.g. soap or not on face, personal toiletries used; religious/cultural beliefs; running water; privacy; gender issues.

Activity Two: Changing the bed linen while the client remains in bed (30 minutes)

The facilitators will demonstrate how to make a bed and change the bottom sheet with a client in bed. Divide the practitioners into small groups of four, each group to practise making a bed. Encourage each practitioner to take it in turns to be the client while the other three practitioners change the bottom sheet with the client in the bed. Remember to ensure that practitioners continue to demonstrate safe patient handling principles. The facilitators should be available in case the practitioners need help.

Questions to Ask Students to Consider while Undertaking this Activity (with Answers)

- What situations can you think of where it would be necessary to change a client's sheet while they are still in bed? – Client is acutely unwell, unable to mobilise or on bed rest, patient transfer from one setting to another and any clients who are bedridden as a result of chronic debilitation.
- When changing the bottom sheet underneath the client why do you want to avoid dragging the sheet out from underneath the client's skin? – This will induce a shearing force that will increase the risk of pressure damage to the client's skin so contributing to the risk of developing pressure ulcers.

Activity Three: Promoting Personal Hygiene and Oral Care of the Client (30 minutes)

The facilitators demonstrate how to give a bed bath to a client who is unable to assist with his/her own care. As the practitioners observe the demonstration, they are encouraged to consider the following questions:
How can practitioners maintain the dignity and privacy of the client?

- Covering with towels, sheets or blankets while being washed reduces the amount of exposure that is necessary

- Preventing other people from entering the room while the client is being washed
- Communicate with the client and observe for non-verbal and verbal cues
- Obtain informed consent by explaining the procedure, ask the clients what they wish to be called and what they want, e.g. soap on face or not, checking temperature of the water frequently, promoting independence.

What can the practitioners learn about the client's activities of daily living while they carry out personal hygiene?

- Independence, dependence of the patient in relation to mobility, hygiene, dressing and continence needs
- Condition of skin and pressure areas
- Pain
- Sleep
- General state of wellbeing
- Psychological and emotional state.

Activity Four: Promoting Personal Hygiene of the Client (60 minutes)

Practitioners to take it in turn to practise assisting with personal hygiene in groups of three. Encourage the client role to give any feedback on the skills of the practitioners.

- One practitioner is the client, one remains in the role of practitioner and one is the observer (practitioners can swop roles so that each person has the opportunity to experience being the practitioner, the client and the observer)
- The practitioner can wash one part of the client's body, for example, face, arm or leg and provide eye care and mouth care.

Ensure that the practitioners consider privacy and dignity within each group. The facilitators are available for help but would only enter the bed space behind the curtains if invited to and permission was sought. If the facilitator can simulate this, it emphasises the importance of privacy and dignity.

- The observer will observe the practitioner and write notes on what the practitioner did well and what could have been improved in relation to: maintaining privacy and dignity, communication and assisting with personal hygiene, eye and mouth care
- The practitioner discusses what he/she thinks went well or could be improved
- The client then gives feedback to the practitioner on his/her experience of being provided with comfort and hygiene. The observer then gives feedback to the practitioner on what went well and what could be improved.

For some practitioners this may be the first time that they have had the opportunity to practise the skill of assisting a client with hygiene needs. When the 'observer' and 'client' are giving feedback to the 'practitioner', make sure that this is done in a constructive and supportive way. The idea is for the practitioners to learn from each other about what went well and where they may need to develop skills and knowledge.

- The practitioner could write comments so that he/she has a record of the self-assessment and peer feedback

- Encourage the practitioner and client to swop roles and repeat until everyone has had a turn at each role and each has had the opportunity to give and receive peer feedback.

Discussion Points and Debrief Points

The following additional theory and learning points could be considered and developed during further discussions, depending on time and the learning needs of the group:

- Why is it important to consider the hygiene needs of our clients? – Personal comfort, dignity and wellbeing of the client to maintain skin, nails and mouth in optimum condition, to prevent infection e.g. mouth care
- Helping a client with their hygiene needs can provide a good opportunity to assess their activities of daily living. What other information can nurses find out about the client while helping them with their hygiene needs? – Independence or dependence of the patient in relation to mobility, hygiene, dressing and continence. Pressure area risk assessment, pain, sleep, general state of wellbeing, nutritional status, emotional status, orientation and cognitive function, and psychosocial circumstances
- Practitioners may consider what risks there are to the client or to themselves while helping a client with their hygiene needs – infection control, e.g. a patient with MRSA or clostridium difficile, moving and handling, the client's risk of falls, risk of developing pressure ulcers (e.g. friction and shear forces when turning client) and allergies (e.g. toiletries, products).

Self-assessment and peer feedback

- What did you think went well and what didn't go well? – please give an explanation
- What feedback did you receive from the client?
- What feedback did you receive from the observer?
- Taking into account your self-assessment and peer feedback, was there anything you would do differently next time? What do you need to learn or practise that will help you to develop your skills of providing comfort and hygiene?

Each clinical activity will require practitioners to have some relevant up-to-date theoretical knowledge, the ability to perform a skill safely and to demonstrate the appropriate professional attitude within their care. Additional reading and reflection of previous skills and experience will allow the practitioners to tailor their learning within the simulation so that it remains relevant and focused.

Some practitioners may already have some experience of the clinical activities relating to personal hygiene, bed bathing and oral care whereas other practitioners may have had no prior experience. In order to assist the facilitators a pre-session self-assessment quiz prior to each clinical skills session would be useful and might be helpful for students to refer to, along with the learning outcomes. This will ensure that the activity remains focused and relevant to the practitioner's learning and within the context of their clinical role.

Table 7.2

Time	Content and Roles	Method	Student Activity	Resources	
10 mins	*Introduction to Session* Lesson aims, link to clinical experiences and discussion of pre-session knowledge and self-assessment	Explanation	Discussion	Toiletries to include flannel, soap, toothbrush and toothpaste	Pre-session activity includes answering questions relating to personal preferences
		Question and answer Discussion	Question and answer		
	Divide students into groups of three – consider prior knowledge and experience of groups so that, if possible, each group has one member who has undertaken healthcare work			Clothing items to include vest top and shorts	
20 mins	*Activity One: Individual Assessment of a Client's Hygiene Needs*	Group work	Group work		
	i In their groups of three or more, practitioners will tell each other one thing that is important to them about their own hygiene regime	Discussion	Discussion		
	ii They will then share their answers to the question: When assessing a client's individual hygiene needs, what factors do you need to consider?				
30 mins (Divide whole group into two if enough facilitators)	*Activity Two: Bed Making – both with/ without a Client in the Bed*	Demonstration of activity	Observation and discussion	Clean linen, pillow cases, blankets, linen skip	
	i Facilitators to demonstrate how to make a bed and how to change a sheet with patient lying on the bed	Simulated practice	Questions to answer in skills book		
	ii Practitioners to practise in small groups of four		Simulated practice		

Time	Content and Roles	Method	Student Activity	Resources	
30 mins	*Activity Three: Assisting with the Comfort and Hygiene Needs of the Client* i The facilitators to demonstrate a full bed bath including eye and oral care ii Practitioners to observe and answer questions	Demonstration and simulation of activity Discussion	Observation Discussion Question and answer Questions to answer	Manikin or volunteer that can be washed and dried Washbowl, soap, flannels, wash cloth, towels Toothbrush, toothpaste, mouthcare tray, sponges, tablets Eye care pack, saline	Ask the practitioners to observe how to maintain privacy and dignity and assess activities of daily living as the facilitator demonstrates the bed bath. They have questions to answer in their skills book relating to this
60 mins	*Activity Four: Assisting with the Comfort and Hygiene Needs of the Client* In groups of three practitioners to practise providing comfort and hygiene including eye and oral care. One student to be the nurse, one the client and one the observer Practitioner to discuss what they think they did well and not so well and then client and observer to feedback to practitioner what went well and not so well. Then swap roles until each have had a turn at being client, practitioner and observer	Simulated practice	Skills practice Peer feedback Self-assessment	As above	The practitioners may feel anxious about being helped to wash, however they should be encouraged to participate in this activity. Advise the practitioners to make sure they consider privacy and dignity within their groups. The facilitators are available for help but will only enter the bed space behind the curtains if invited to do so. It is useful to make the link between the practitioner's anxiety at

(Continued)

Table 7.2 (Continued)

Time	Content and Roles	Method	Student Activity	Resources
				being washed and the client's experience when being assisted with their hygiene needs
				The practitioners are asked to feedback to each other so advise them to be constructive and supportive when giving feedback
10 mins	*Summary* Including time to complete any remaining questions and expand on related activities that can be rehearsed			

FURTHER READING

Department of Health (2010) *Essence of Care Benchmarks for the Fundamental Aspects of Care. Benchmarks for Personal Hygiene.* London: DH.
The benchmarks relevant to this session include:
Benchmark for personal and oral hygiene.
Benchmarks for privacy and dignity.
Benchmarks for principles of self-care.

REFERENCES

Baillie, L. (ed.) (2005) *Developing Practical Skills*, 2nd edn. London: Hodder Arnold.

Benbow, M. (2008) 'Pressure ulcer prevention and pressure relieving surfaces', *British Journal of Nursing*, 17 (13): 830–5.

Department of Health (2010) *Essence of Care 2010. Benchmarks for the fundamental aspects of care. Benchmarks for Personal Hygiene.* London. Department of Health. Available on: http://www.dh.gov.uk/en/Publicationsandstatistics/Publications/Publications PolicyAndGuidance/DH_4005475 [accessed 19 April 2011].

Downey, L. and Lloyd, H. (2008) 'Bed bathing patients in hospital', *Nursing Standard*, 22 (34): 35–40.

Evans, G. (2001) 'A rationale for oral care', *Nursing Standard*, 15 (43): 33–6.

Kozier, B., Erb, G., Berman, A., Snyder, S., Lake, R. and Harvey, S. (2009) *Fundamentals of Nursing, Concepts, Process and Practice.* London: Pearson Education.

Malkin, B. and Berridge, P. (2009) 'Guidance on maintaining personal hygiene in nail care', *Nursing Standard*, 23 (41): 35–8.

National Institute for Clinical Excellence (NICE) (2005) *The Prevention and Treatment of Pressure Ulcers.* London: NICE. Available on: http://www.nice.org.uk [accessed 19 April 2011].

Nursing Times Clinical (2003) 'NT skills update – eye care', *Nursing Times*, 99: 8.

Pegram, A., Bloomfield, J. and Jones, A. (2007) 'Clinical skills: bed bathing and personal hygiene needs of patients', *British Journal of Nursing*, 16 (6): 356–8.

Xavier, G. (2000) 'The importance of mouth care in preventing infection', *Nursing Standard*, 14 (18): 47–51.

8

ELIMINATION: URINALYSIS, BOWEL CARE AND CATHETER CARE

Alison Eddleston

Aim

The aim of this chapter is to facilitate the development of healthcare skills by exploring the knowledge and skills needed to support catheter care, urinalysis and bowel care in a variety of clinical and simulation environments.

Objectives

On completion of this chapter you will be able to:

- Review the underpinning knowledge needed to support the acquisition of healthcare skills in relation to:
  - Catheter care
  - Urinalysis
  - Bowel care
- Explain and demonstrate the clinical procedures needed to support the development of the named clinical skills:

- Catheter care
- Urinalysis
- Bowel care

- Explore the use of simulation in order to enhance clinical skill acquisition.

INTRODUCTION TO THE SKILL

Many people receive healthcare that is effective and appropriate to their needs and preferences. However, practice and care is not always correct and, therefore, improvements need to be made (DH, 2010). The development of healthcare skills is needed in order to ensure safe and competent practice is delivered by both healthcare educators and students.

Catheter care, urinalysis and bowel care are three key areas which are needed in order to assist a person with the process of elimination. Developing clinical skills in these areas is fundamental in determining which interventions are needed to ensure that this essential care is given with knowledge and competence (Walker, 2009). The use of both clinical skills equipment and simulation technology can enable the above clinical skills to be developed in a supportive environment.

BACKGROUND TO THE SKILL

Elimination of urine and faeces is an essential bodily function that most of us perform without much thought and is a natural process critical for human functioning (Evans-Smith, 2005, cited by Walker, 2009). This is until this process becomes either disrupted or hindered by acute illness, altered physiology, or the dependence on others for support and care.

In order to support the elimination process, you will need to be able to develop or enhance your physical and psychological healthcare skills. This is because both catheter and bowel care require you to develop discretion, patience and understanding as well as providing both personal and intimate care.

GETTING READY TO PERFORM THE SKILL

PROFESSIONAL RESPONSIBILITY

In order to meet the needs of a person's catheter and bowel care, you are required to apply a level of knowledge and provide a rationale and evidence base for your actions (Walker, 2009). This requires both the healthcare educator and student to ensure they can access evidence-based information in order to ensure that bladder and bowel care is tailored to an individual's need and preferences in an environment appropriate to their needs (Department of Health (DH), 2010).

Regular exposure to the healthcare skills involved in bladder and bowel care is essential in either gaining or maintaining the necessary knowledge and skills (Nursing and Midwifery Council (NMC), 2008). As you are personally accountable for your own practice, it is your responsibility to ensure you have the necessary knowledge and skills to provide the care needed (NMC, 2008). However, if an aspect of practice is beyond your level of competence, you must obtain the necessary help and supervision from a competent practitioner until you acquire the requisite knowledge and skills (Cairns, 2011).

You will also be required to benchmark your standards of care to both local and national guidelines. This to ensure that once you have developed your own professional knowledge and skills your clinical competence is measured against evidence-based care pathways and protocols (Department of Health (DH), 2010). This can be achieved by ensuring the elements of the care process are delivered by exploring key policies, procedures and audit (Department of Health (DH), 2006).

AWARENESS OF KEY ANATOMY AND PHYSIOLOGY INVOLVED IN THE URINARY AND GASTROINTESTINAL SYSTEMS

As discussed, it is important to be able to recognise abnormal or altered physiological changes that may have occurred in the process of elimination. Therefore it is fundamental that you explore the normal physiological processes within the urinary system, in order that you are able to identify potential problems or issues (Lawson and Peate, 2009). Recognition of normal anatomy and physiological processes within the urinary system will enhance the development of the healthcare skills needed with regards to both catheter care and urinalysis.

Key areas to review:

- Anatomical structures – kidneys, ureter, bladder, urethra
- Process of micturition.

Likewise it is essential that you also develop an understanding of the process of digestion and review how it is affected by the different components of the gastrointestinal tract (Lawson and Peate, 2009). This is necessary in order to be able to assess for abnormal function or problems associated with digestion or gastrointestinal disease.

Key areas to review:

- Anatomical structures – sigmoid colon, rectum
- Process of digestion.

PATIENT ASSESSMENT

Once you have explored the key anatomy and physiology involved in the process of elimination, it is essential to consider individual assessment needs. The process of assessment comprises two key areas, namely clinical history taking and the examination process. It is also important to note that, while the urinary system and gastrointestinal tract are two distinct systems, similarities exist with regards to the information required from both systems. This is because the impact of one system's problems may be demonstrated in another system. For example, an individual who has had a low fluid and nutritional intake may experience low urine output and this may also be demonstrated by an altered bowel habit such as constipation due to inadequate fluid intake.

The first area to explore is the history of events; this will enable you to develop some insight and understanding into any issues or problems that may have occurred. This information can be developed further to identify any normal patterns of behaviour with regards to urinary and bowel habits. Another key area as discussed above is dietary and fluid intake, which needs to be assessed along with any medication history to identify any potential issues that require management.

Once you have gathered the above information and identified any issues or problems, you are then able to consider how these issues may impact on the physical examination and care process. The examination process is vital as it allows for the inspection of the external genitalia with respect to anatomical differences and abnormalities that may be present from both a gender and altered disease perspective. Key areas to review include the anatomical positioning of the urethral meatus; this is particular important in maintaining personal hygiene and providing catheter care. The external genitalia can then be inspected for signs of infection, inflammation and excoriation.

Bowel elimination is a sensitive issue and requires effective care and management (Dougherty and Lister, 2008). The physical examination allows the key anatomical structures involved to be examined in order to establish the appropriate care required. As discussed previously, key structures may have been altered by a disease process; therefore it is essential that the anal area is observed for signs of infection, inflammation and excoriation as well as any abnormalities.

Some patients who have had bowel surgery may have had bowel or urinary stoma formed from a section of bowel that has been brought out on to the abdominal wall (Dougherty and Lister, 2008). This will require specialist management and, therefore, further advice and support needs to be sought prior to care delivery. Also, with regard to rectal function, it is important to be aware of whether the rectum is functioning or non-functioning following surgery.

Once the above information has been considered, it is important to obtain patient consent so that individualised examination and care may be delivered following this information gathering process.

CONSENT

It is a general legal and ethical principle that valid consent must be obtained before starting any treatment, physical investigation or providing personal care (Department of Health (DH), 2009). It is also essential to be aware that prior to obtaining consent, you need to ensure a person has the capacity to make an informed choice about their care process. This is because the capacity to consent may be temporarily hindered due to the effects of trauma, illness or medication (Department of Health (DH), 2009).

The Mental Capacity Act Code of Practice (Department of Health (DH), 2005) sets forth a framework to protect people who lack the capacity to make such decisions. In order for consent to be valid, it needs to be given voluntarily and without duress or harm. An individual may give their consent verbally or non-verbally and this is evident through their actions. However, it may also be necessary on occasions to seek written consent as an individual may need a procedure at a later date.

If a healthcare professional does not respect the legal and ethical principles involved in consent, they may be liable to legal action both by the patient or their professional body (Department of Health (DH), 2009).

DOCUMENTATION

The Department of Health introduced national benchmarks in 2001 to ensure that essential care was structured and patient focussed. The essence of care benchmarks became general indicators for best practice and provided a framework for health-care practitioners to compare patient care. These indicators of best practice have ensured that bladder and bowel care remains a fundamental aspect of essential care (Department of Health (DH), 2010).

Additional political initiatives have also resulted in the drive to ensure individualised evidence-based practice and care. Examples which support both catheter and bladder care include: *Essential Steps to Safe Clean Care* (Department of Health (DH), 2006) and *Saving Lives: Reducing Infection, Delivering Clean and Safe Care* (DH, 2007). It is important to develop knowledge of these initiatives in order to deliver and document continuing catheter and bowel care. It is essential that the documentation of care provides both an evidence base and a record of the care or continuing care to be given.

PROCEDURE

CATHETER CARE

Catheter care is the essential continuing care required to maintain the integrity of an indwelling urinary catheter that has been inserted using skilled aseptic technique into the urethral meatus (Pratt and Pellowe, 2010). Approximately one in four hospitalised patients will require a urinary catheter at some time during their stay and at least 7% of these patients will develop a healthcare associated infection as a result of urinary catheterisation (Odell, 2007).

Healthcare educators and students need to become familiar with essential elements of this continuing care process and the equipment required in order to ensure safe

Table 8.1

Elements of Continuing Care	Equipment Required
Catheter assessment – the need for urinary catheterisation	Continuing care bundle
Catheter review – size, length, balloon, drainage system	Documentation Policy/guidelines Patient records
Prevention of healthcare-associated infection – hand and catheter hygiene	Personal protective equipment Disposable gloves Apron Eye/face protection Disposable bowl Wipes Soap solution Clinical waste bag
Maintaining integrity of the urinary drainage system	Appropriate sterile drainage collection bag for patient need Holder or stand for drainage bag
Urine sampling	Sampling container Sterile receiver Jug Selection of swabs saturated with 70% isopropyl alcohol

Action	Rationale
Explain to the patient the procedure and the continuing catheter care that is needed	To ensure that the patient understands the procedure and has the mental capacity to provide valid consent (Dougherty and Lister, 2008)
Provide the patient with any written information such as information leaflets or booklets	The patient should be fully informed about the procedure and therefore education should begin following insertion and provide an outline to the patient of catheter care required (Robinson, 2006; Pratt and Pellowe, 2010)
Prepare the environment ready for the procedure to occur by screening the surrounding area with privacy screens/curtains	To provide privacy and maintain patient dignity throughout the care process
Gather and collect the equipment and relevant local policies and guidelines needed for the procedure of catheter care	To document the care episode provided

(Continued)

Table 8.1   (Continued)

Elements of Continuing Care	Equipment Required
Arrange the equipment in the working environment. This may be a cleaned bedside trolley or area in the healthcare environment	To ensure the environment is safe for the healthcare practitioner to provide the care needed
Support the patient into the required position for the care to be performed	To maintain safe positioning and patient safety throughout the procedure
Wash hands using the correct hand hygiene procedure	To decontaminate hands prior to patient contact in order to reduce the risk of a healthcare associated infection (DH, 2007)
Apply the appropriate personal protective equipment. For example, disposable gloves, apron and face protection if needed	To reduce the risk of cross infection (Dougherty and Lister, 2008)
Inspect the external genitalia and review the urethra meatus in order to observe the catheter entry site	The external genitalia area needs to be inspected for anatomical positioning, signs of infection, inflammation, excoriation, discharge, bleeding and over granulation (RCN, 2008)
Review the catheter and document the following areas: • Size – 12–14 Ch is generally sufficient for both men and women. Size 16–18 Ch should only be used if there is debris present (Cairns, 2011)	To ensure patients have the smallest size catheter to meet their needs (RCN, 2008)
• Length – A standard length catheter also known as a male is 40–45cm. whilst a female length being 20–26cm (NSPA, 2009, cited by Pomfret, 2010)	To ensure the correct length of catheter has been inserted to prevent trauma and even death due to anatomical urethral differences due to gender (RCN, 2008; Pomfret, 2010)
• Balloon size – Should be no greater than 10 millilitres	Avoids catheter-associated problems of pressure damage to the neck of the bladder and catheter bypassing problems (Head, 2006; Robinson, 2006)
Clean the catheter site as per local policy (DH, 2007). Cleaning the urethral meatus is demonstrated in Figure 8.1.	To minimise the risk of infection of the urinary tract. Avoid vigorous meatal cleaning with antiseptic solutions (Dougherty and Lister, 2008)

Elements of Continuing Care	Equipment Required
Make sure the patient is comfortable following catheter cleansing and ensure the urethral area is dry	If the area is left wet or moist, secondary infection may result (Dougherty and Lister, 2008)
Select a sterile closed urinary drainage system appropriate to the patient clinical need. For example, hourly measurement, volume control, leg/night bag (Head, 2006)	To prevent the spread of infection healthcare practitioners should ensure the connection between the drainage system is not broken except for clinical need (DH, 2006)
Position the drainage system on a holder or stand above floor level but below bladder level	To prevent reflux or contamination (DH, 2006, 2007) and support patient comfort (Dougherty and Lister, 2008)
Obtain a urine sample if needed from the sampling port using an aseptic non-touch technique	
Empty the urinary drainage bag often and as necessary	To maintain urinary flow and prevent reflux (Pratt and Pellowe, 2010)
Dispose of any urine and equipment following the care episode according to local policies and guidelines	To prevent the spread of infection (DH, 2006)
Wash hands using the correct hand hygiene procedure	To decontaminate hands prior to patient contact in order to reduce the risk of a healthcare associated infection (DH, 2007)
Record and document the care episode according to local policy and guidelines	To ensure effective documented care that is consistent, reliable and evidence focussed
Following the procedure ensure the patient is comfortable and provide any further information that may be required	To ensure the patient is fully informed of the care given and the need to prevent urinary tract infection (Pratt and Pellowe, 2010)

and effective care is given that reduces the incidence of a healthcare-associated infection as a result of urinary catheterisation (Department of Health (DH), 2006, 2007; Royal College of Nursing (RCN), 2008).

URINALYSIS

Urinalysis is the testing of the physical characteristics and composition of freshly voided urine (Dougherty and Lister, 2007). Urine is characteristically pale to deep

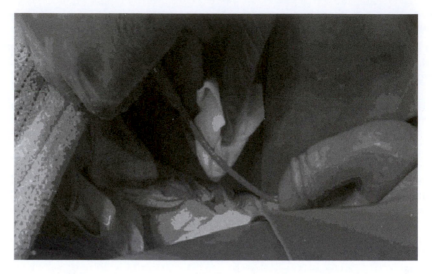

Figure 8.1

yellow in colour and is slightly acidic; however, the colour and composition of urine can change dramatically as a result of illness and disease (Dougherty and Lister, 2008).

Urinalysis can provide both a baseline measurement and be utilised as a diagnostic tool in order to assess for normal and abnormal substances present in the composition of urine (Steggall, 2007; Dougherty and Lister, 2008). It is also an important part of patient assessment which could indicate the presence of a serious disease or guide a patient's future management (Steggall, 2007).

BOWEL CARE

Bowel elimination is a basic bodily function that most people carry out in private and are often embarrassed to discuss publicly (Pellatt, 2007). As normal bowel habits vary from one person to another it is hard to arrive at a single definition (Kyle, 2007). There appear to be three key problems associated with bowel dysfunction, these are referred to as faecal incontinence, diarrhoea and constipation.

In order to overcome such problems, bowel care needs to be specific to the individual and problems associated with the dysfunction. This requires an individual evidence-based care pathway to be developed that takes into account both personal needs and preferences (DH, 2010). This is particularly important for patients who have received a spinal cord injury as a specialised protocol will be required which considers the nature and impact of the spinal injury.

Table 8.2

Elements of Urinalysis	Equipment Required
Urine sampling	Sampling container Sterile receiver Catheter specimen Selection of swabs saturated with 70% isopropyl alcohol
Urinalysis	Urine specimen Urine reagent sticks Documentation
Prevention of healthcare-associated infection – hand and catheter hygiene	Personal protective equipment Disposable gloves Apron Eye/face protection Clinical waste bag

Action	Rationale
Explain to the patient the procedure and the need for urinalysis	To ensure that the patient understands the procedure and has the mental capacity to provide valid consent (Dougherty and Lister, 2008)
Provide the patient with any written information such as information leaflets or booklets	The patient should be fully informed about the procedure and receive appropriate counselling if further results are needed (Steggall, 2007)
Prepare the environment ready for the patient either to provide a urine sample or screen the surrounding area with privacy screens/curtains to obtain a catheter sample	To provide privacy and maintain patient dignity throughout the care process
Gather and collect the equipment and relevant local policies and guidelines needed for the procedure of catheter care	To document the care episode provided
Arrange the equipment in the working environment. This may be at the bedside or area in the healthcare environment	To ensure the environment is safe for the healthcare practitioner to perform urinalysis
Wash hands using the correct hand hygiene procedure	To decontaminate hands prior to patient contact in order to reduce the risk of a healthcare associated infection (DH, 2007)

(Continued)

Table 8.2   (Continued)

Action	Rationale
Apply the appropriate personal protective equipment. For example, disposable gloves, apron and face protection if needed	To reduce the risk of cross infection (Dougherty and Lister, 2008)
Obtain a clean urine sample from either the patient or the catheter sampling port using an aseptic non-touch technique	Urine that has been stored deteriorates rapidly and can give false results (Dougherty and Lister, 2008)
Observe the sample of urine for: • Colour • Concentration • Odour • Presence of particles (Nicol et al., 2004)	To assess for normal characteristics and identify any abnormalities
Fully immerse the reagent strip into the urine and remove immediately and tap against the side of the container	To remove excess urine (Dougherty and Lister, 2008)
Wait the required time interval before reading the strip against the colour chart (see Figure 8.2)	The strip must be read at exactly the time interval specified or the reagents will not have time to react or may be inaccurate (Dougherty and Lister, 2008)
Document your findings in relation to: • Specific gravity(SG) • pH • Protein • Blood • Glucose • Ketones • Urobilinogen and biliruben • Leucocytes • Nitrite (Steggall, 2007)	To assess for normal composition and identify any abnormalities
Dispose of any urine and equipment following the care episode using local policies and guidelines	To prevent the risk of healthcare associated infection (DH, 2007)
Wash hands using the correct hand hygiene procedure	To decontaminate hands prior to patient contact in order to reduce the risk of a healthcare associate infection (DH, 2007)

Action	Rationale
Record and document the care episode according to local policy and guidelines	To ensure effective documented care that is consistent, reliable and evidence focussed
Following the procedure ensure the patient is comfortable and provide any further information that may be required	To ensure the patient is fully informed of the care given and the need to prevent urinary tract infection (Pratt and Pellowe, 2010)

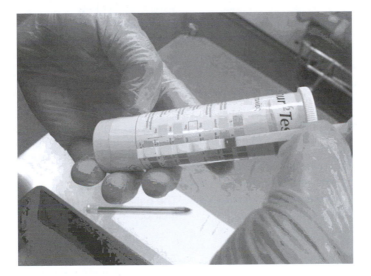

Figure 8.2

Healthcare educators and students need to develop the underpinning knowledge in relation to the assessment of bowel function and the medicine management required to correct bowel dysfunction. Both rectal suppositories and enemas are medications that can be given via the rectal route to produce local or systemic effects and correct bowel dysfunction. However, particular care is required in relation to the intimate nature of the procedures needed to manage care delivery (Pegram et al., 2008).

POINTS TO NOTE

As a healthcare educator it is important that you consider your own level of underpinning knowledge as well as your exposure to the healthcare skills associated with catheter care, urinalysis and bowel care. This is required to ensure you have the competence to ensure safe competent practice is delivered.

It is essential that you also explore the key issues of consent with healthcare students as this may be their first exposure to gaining verbal or non-verbal consent

Table 8.3

Elements of Bowel Care	Equipment Required
Bowel assessment – the need for bowel care and management	Documentation Policy/guidelines Patient records
Prevention of healthcare-associated infection – hand and catheter hygiene	Personal protective equipment Disposable gloves Apron Eye/face protection Clinical waste bag
Maintaining integrity of the bowel function Stool sample Administration of rectal medication suppositories/enema	Stool sample container Suppositories Enema Lubricate Swabs

Action	Rationale
Explain to the patient the procedure and the continuing bowel care that is needed	To ensure that the patient understands the procedure and has the mental capacity to provide valid consent (Dougherty and Lister, 2008)
Provide the patient with any written information such as information leaflets or booklets	The patient should be fully informed about their bowel care needs (DH, 2010)
Prepare the environment ready for the procedure to occur by screening the surrounding area with privacy screens/curtains	To provide privacy and maintain patient dignity throughout the care process
Gather and collect the equipment and relevant local policies and guidelines needed for the procedure of catheter care	To document the care episode provided
Arrange the equipment in the working environment. This may be a cleaned bedside trolley or area in the healthcare environment	To ensure the environment is safe for the healthcare practitioner to provide the care needed
Wash hands using the correct hand hygiene procedure	To decontaminate hands prior patient contact in order to reduce the risk of a healthcare associated infection (DH, 2007)

Action	Rationale

Apply the appropriate personal protective equipment. For example, disposable gloves, apron and face protection if needed	To reduce the risk of cross infection (Dougherty and Lister, 2008)

Obtain a stool sample if needed by assisting the patient to use a bedpan/ commode and observe the faeces for:
 	
   Amount
   Frequency
   Consistency
   Colour
   Pain/discomfort
   Flatus
   (Nicol et al., 2004)
	To assess and observe bowel function

Support the patient into the required position for the care to be performed. Lie the patient on the left hand side with the knees flexed. Place an incontinence pad under the patient and cover to maintain dignity (Dougherty and Lister, 2008)	This allows ease of passage into the rectum by following the natural anatomy of the colon (Dougherty and Lister, 2008)
Inspect the anal area	The anal area needs assessing for anatomical positioning, signs of infection, inflammation, excoriation, discharge, rectal bleeding, haemorrhoids and skin tags (Pegram et al., 2008)
Administration of Enema if Required	
Warm the enema to the manufacturer's instructions	To aid ease of administration and prevent distension and discomfort (Dougherty and Lister, 2008)
Lubricate nozzle of enema and expel any air Introduce the nozzle to a depth of 10–12.5 cm while parting the buttocks. Squeeze the enema into the rectum from the base container.	To ensure maximum effect if constipation present (Pegram et al., 2008)
Action	**Rationale**

(Continued)

Table 8.3   (Continued)

Ask the patient to hold as long as possible	
Administration of Suppositories if required	
Lubricate the end of the suppository and insert into the anal canal to a depth of 2–4 cm. Repeat a second time if necessary	Allows the lower edge of the rectal sphincter to close around the rectum (Dougherty and Lister, 2008)
Clean the rectal and perianal area as per local policy. Make sure the patient is comfortable following rectal review	If the area is left wet or moist secondary infection may result (Dougherty and Lister, 2008).
Dispose of any faeces and equipment following the care episode using local policies and guidelines.	
Wash hands using the correct hand hygiene procedure.	To decontaminate hands prior to patient contact in order to reduce the risk of a healthcare associate infection (DH, 2007)
Record and document the care episode according to local policy and guidelines	To ensure effective documented care that is consistent, reliable and evidence focussed
Following the procedure ensure the patient is comfortable and provide any further information that may be required	To ensure the patient is fully informed of the care given

for such an intimate or personal procedure. It is also paramount for healthcare students to be aware that consent may be given but that it may also be withdrawn at any point in the care delivery process.

A key area that also needs to be explored is regarding the professional responsibilities of the healthcare student and practitioner when performing the skills. This is particularly important due to the intimate nature of care required. A key issue to discuss is gender and its implications for clinical practice, e.g. a female practitioner performing catheter care on a male patient and, likewise, a male practitioner performing catheter care on a female patient.

The healthcare educator also needs to ensure that they are familiar with any local Trust policies and guidelines with regard to cleaning solutions, equipment and key documentation utilised. This will ensure that the healthcare skills session meets current local clinical practice.

CONCLUSION

Within this chapter the healthcare skills associated with catheter care, urinalysis and bowel care have been discussed. This has been achieved by reviewing the underpinning knowledge needed to perform the healthcare skills and exploring the procedures involved in continuing catheter care, urinalysis and bowel care.

Developing healthcare skills in these three areas is fundamental in determining which interventions are needed to ensure that this essential care is given with knowledge and competence (Walker, 2009). The use of the simulation scenario has been designed to develop your own healthcare skills further by ensuring competent practice is developed in a safe and secure environment.

HOW TO USE SIMULATION TO TEACH THE SKILL

Introduction

This simulation scenario has been designed to explore and demonstrate the healthcare skills needed to deliver continuing catheter care in a healthcare environment.

Learning Objectives

By the end of this scenario the healthcare professional will be able to:

- Review the elements involved in continuing catheter care
- Discuss and collect the appropriate equipment needed prior to the procedure of catheter care
- Demonstrate the procedure of catheter care using a simulation manikin
- Evaluate the simulation experience identifying an area of personal learning.

Resources

Equipment

- Simulation manikin suitable for urinary catheterisation with a size 12 Ch urinary catheter in situ with a 10 ml balloon

SIMULATION SCENARIO

- Key documentation:

  - Policy/guidelines
  - Patient records

- Personal protective equipment:

  - Disposable gloves
  - Apron
  - Eye/face protection

- Disposable bowl, wipes, soap solution, clinical waste bag
- Appropriate drainage collection bag for patient need
- Holder or stand for drainage bag.

Setting

This scenario could be performed in a clinical skills laboratory or a simulated area within a healthcare setting.

Time Element

There is no designated time limit for this simulation session; however, it is important to ensure the time for the skill to be performed ensures safe and competent practice.

Scenario

Jean is a 76-year-old lady who has been admitted to your clinical area following a bowel perforation with faecal peritonitis due to caecal carcinoma. Jean is fully conscious and orientated to her surroundings.

   As part of her continuing care needs, you are requested to deliver Jean's continuing catheter care. Prior to the procedure one of the healthcare students asks if she can assist you with this procedure.

Role of Participants

Healthcare Practitioner

Discuss the elements of the continuing catheter care listed below with the healthcare student:

- Catheter assessment – the need for urinary catheterisation
- Catheter review – size, length, balloon, drainage system Prevention of healthcare associated infection – hand and catheter hygiene
- Maintaining integrity of the urinary drainage system.

Perform the elements of the continuing catheter care required on the simulation manikin.

Healthcare Student

Evaluate the continuing catheter care given.
Identify an area of personal learning.

Areas for Discussion and Debrief Technique

Healthcare Practitioner

Individual discussion and feedback exploring healthcare skills technique from:

- Healthcare educator
- Healthcare student.

Consider the use of video technology to support the analysis and visual feedback of the dialogue and catheter care given.

Healthcare Student

This is an opportunity for individual discussion with and questions to the healthcare practitioner, exploring healthcare skills techniques.

If used, review the video of the simulation to support the analysis and visual feedback of the dialogue between the patient, healthcare student and practitioner.

Points for Consideration

- Patient consent
- Communication process
- The continuing catheter care procedure and skills required
- Any areas for future professional learning and development.

REFERENCES

Cairns, P. (2011) 'Urinary catheterisation', unpublished, University of Central Lancashire.

Department of Health (DH) (2001) *The Essence of Care: Patient-focussed Benchmarking for Healthcare Practitioners*. London: Department of Health.

Department of Health (2005) *Mental Capacity Act 2005 Code of Practice*. London: Department of Health.

Department of Health (2006) *Essential Steps to Safe, Clean Care*. London: Department of Health.

Department of Health (2007) *Saving Lives: Reducing Infection, Delivering Clean and Safe Care*. London: Department of Health.

Department of Health (2009) *Reference Guide to Consent for Examination or Treatment*, 2nd edn. London: Department of Health.

Department of Health (2010) *Essence of Care 2010 Benchmarks for Care Environment*. London: Department of Health.

Dougherty, L. and Lister, S. (2008) *The Royal Marsden Hospital Manual of Clinical Nursing Procedures*, Student Edition. Oxford: Wiley & Sons Ltd.

Head, C. (2006) 'Insertion of a urinary catheter', *Nursing Older People*, 18 (10): 33–6.

Kyle, G. (2007) 'Bowel care part 1 – assessment of constipation', *Nursing Times*, 103 (42): 26–7.

Lawson, L. and Peate, I. (2009) *Essential Nursing Care A Workbook For Clinical Practice.* Chichester: Wiley & Sons.

Nicol, M., Bavin, C., Bedford-Turner, S., Cronin, P. and Rawlings-Anderson, K. (2004) *Essential Nursing Skills*, 2nd edn. London: Elsevier Limited.

Nursing and Midwifery Council (2008) *The Code Standards of Conduct, Performance and Ethics for Nurses and Midwives.* London: NMC.

Odell, M. (2007) 'NHS research evaluates treated catheters', *British Association of Critical Care Nurses, Nursing in Critical Care*, 12 (5): 255.

Pegram, A., Blookfield, J. and Jones, A. (2008) 'Safe use of rectal suppositories and enemas with adult patients', *Nursing Standard*, 22 (38): 38–40.

Pellatt, G.C. (2007) 'Clinical skills: bowel elimination and management of complications', *British Journal of Nursing*, 16 (6): 351–5.

Pomfret, I. (2010) 'Catheter care: is it really improving?' *Journal of Community Nursing*, 24 (5): 26–8.

Pratt, R. and Pellowe, C. (2010) 'Good practice in management of patients with urethral catheters', *Nursing Older People*, 22 (8): 25–9.

Robinson, J. (2006) 'Selecting a urinary catheter and drainage system', *British Journal of Nursing*, 15 (19): 1045–50.

Royal College of Nursing (RCN) (2008) *Catheter Care RCN Guidance for Nurses.* London: RCN.

Steggall, M.J. (2007) 'Urine samples and urinalysis', *Nursing Standard*, 22 (14–16): 42–5.

Walker, S.H. (2009) 'Continence, bowel and bladder care', in H. Iggulden, C. Macdonald, and K. Staniland (eds), *Clinical Skills: The Essence of Caring.* London: Open University Press. Chapter 10.

9

NUTRITION: FEEDING A PATIENT, FLUID BALANCE AND NASOGASTRIC FEEDING

Kim Harley and Helen Holder

Aim

The aim of this chapter is to give an overview of the principles of the procedure to pass a fine bore feeding tube and its aftercare, with reference to monitoring, potential complications and maintenance of hydration and nutrition.

Objectives

- Discuss indications and contraindications to nasogastric feeding tube insertion
- Describe the correct procedure for fine bore nasogastric feeding tube insertion
- Identify the key issues surrounding management of the patient with a nasogastric feeding tube and enteral feed.

INTRODUCTION TO THE SKILL AND EXPLANATION OF ITS IMPORTANCE

Enteral tube feeding (ETF) is used to feed patients who have an inadequate oral intake from food and/or oral nutritional supplements, or who cannot eat/drink safely (National Institute for Clinical Excellence (NICE), 2006). Nasogastric (NG) feeding is the most common first line approach to short-term ETF, providing direct access to the stomach if a patient's oral intake is inadequate or contraindicated (Best, 2005; 2007; NICE, 2006; May, 2007). However, occasionally a NG tube (NGT) can be used for long-term feeding where insertion of an alternative long-term enteral tube is not indicated or tolerated (Roberts, 2007). An NGT may also be used to facilitate gastric drainage (Dougherty and Lister, 2008).

An NG feeding tube is inserted via the nose and oesophagus into the stomach and is relatively easy to place by a skilled nurse/healthcare practitioner (Endacott et al., 2009). The skill of NG tube insertion is, therefore, important as a delay in the provision of nutritional support can lead to an increased risk or worsening of malnutrition and a subsequent deterioration in the patient's condition (NICE, 2006). Furthermore, Horsburgh et al. (2008) highlighted that skilled NG tube insertion is important to patients, practitioners and relatives and that current training may be insufficient, particularly in caring for patients with complex needs such as dysphagic stroke patients. This chapter therefore aims to provide a guide to NG insertion to support the development of this skill in clinical practice in accordance with local policies and procedures.

BACKGROUND TO THE SKILL

It is important to assess and identify patients who are malnourished or at risk of worsening malnutrition on admission to hospital in order to plan effective nutritional care. Malnutrition is still prevalent in hospitals and the community, with recent evidence of at least one third of patients being identified as malnourished on admission to hospital and during their hospital stay (British Association of Parenteral and Enteral Nutrition (BAPEN), 2009). Therefore it is recommended that nutritional screening is carried out on all patients on admission to hospital, using a valid and reliable nutritional screening tool such as the Malnutrition Universal Screening Tool (MUST) (Malnutrition Advisory Group, 2003) (NICE, 2006). A score is calculated which then indicates if a patient requires further observation and/or nutritional assessment and provision of nutritional support such as NG feeding.

INDICATIONS FOR NASOGASTRIC FEEDING

The decision to initiate an enteral tube feed depends on several factors such as the patient's diagnosis, function of the gastrointestinal (GI) tract, length of time nutritional support is required, resources available and the patient's preference. However, NG feeding is still considered the first choice for enteral nutritional support as it is generally easy to initiate and discontinue once oral intake has been re-established. It is, therefore, indicated in patients who require short-term enteral feeding and have a functional gastrointestinal tract without complications such as vomiting or aspiration (Bowling, 2004: 43; Best, 2007). Examples of conditions that may require nasogastric feeding are illustrated in Table 9.1.

Table 9.1

Indications for Nasogastric Feeding	Example
Impaired swallow/dysphagia	Stroke, multiple sclerosis, motor neurone disease, Parkinson's disease, head injury
Altered consciousness	Ventilated patients and those for whom oral feeding is not possible
Increased nutritional requirements	Cancer, sepsis, liver disease, HIV, cystic fibrosis, burns, inflammatory bowel disease
Incomplete orophayngeal/oesophageal obstruction	Head and neck cancer, oesophageal cancer
Supplementary feeding	Gut dysmobility or short intestinal length
Psychological problems	Severe depression and anorexia nervosa

Sources: Bowling, 2004: 43; NICE, 2006

The National Institute for Clinical Excellence (NICE) (2006) recommend that patients with dysphagia are given a two- to four-week trial of nasogastric feeding and that gastrostomy feeding should be considered in patients who are likely to need ETF for greater than four weeks.

CONTRAINDICATIONS TO NASOGASTRIC FEEDING

NG feeding may not be suitable for all patients as illustrated in Table 9.2.

Table 9.2

Contraindications to Nasogastric Feeding	Rationale
Inaccessible upper GI tract e.g. obstructive head and neck and oesophageal tumours	Preventing passage of the NG tube into the stomach
Gastro-oesophageal reflux, poor gastric emptying, ileus and intestinal obstruction	Increasing risk of aspiration of gastric contents and poor absorption of nutrients
Proximal GI tract fistula, facial injury and cervical spine injury (suspected or confirmed)	Risk of NG tube displacement on insertion

Sources: Bowling, 2004: 43; NICE, 2006

Care should be taken when inserting NGTs in patients with a pharyngeal or oesophageal pouch and oesophageal varices to avoid potential perforation or rupture (Best, 2007). Advice should be sought from the referring medical or surgical team before attempting blind insertion in such patients.

Patients who have an inaccessible upper gastrointestinal tract or are at risk of aspiration, such as gastric outlet obstruction, should be considered for post pyloric feeding (Bowling, 2004: 43; NICE, 2006).

GETTING READY TO PERFORM THE SKILLS

PRIOR KNOWLEDGE OF LEARNERS

Students need knowledge of the anatomy and physiology of the upper GI tract and the respiratory tract, including the nasopharynx, oropharynx and larngopharynx, as this is a common passageway for food and water, and air passage in and out of the lungs (Colbert et al., 2009: 411). Therefore, a prior knowledge of the physiology of swallowing is also required to prevent inadvertent tube placement into the lungs and prevent complications once feeding is established.

Knowledge of the pathophysiology of the upper GI tract and respiratory tract is also required in order to assess the patient's suitability for NG feeding.

Informed consent should be obtained before attempting NG tube insertion as follows:

- The procedure/method of nutritional support should be explained in terms that the patient can understand, with regard for any communication difficulties
- Consent can be verbal, written or implied, depending on the nature of the procedure, although verbal or implied is usually sufficient for NGT insertion. Refusal is binding in the competent person
- Patients who lack capacity must remain at the centre of decision making and are fully safeguarded
- Where the patient is not competent to make a decision, an attempt at the procedure can be made if it is considered to be in the client's best interests. (Mental Capacity Act 2005; NICE, 2006; NMC, 2008; DH, 2009; RCP, 2010)

Generally the decision to start an enteral tube feed is made in conjunction with the patient, carer and multidisciplinary team. It is usually considered to be appropriate when the therapeutic aim is to improve or maintain physical condition, that is, where the benefit outweighs the burden. However, it may be inappropriate when the aim is palliative, and comfort and symptom relief are the priority. Tube feeding may also be withheld if the perceived burden outweighs probable benefit, although a time trial of tube feeding is recommended where the outcome is uncertain (British Medical Association (BMA), 2007; Royal College of Physicians (RCP), 2010).

TUBE SELECTION AND OTHER EQUIPMENT WITH RATIONALE FOR CHOICE

For the purpose of NG feeding, a fine bore feeding tube is used (Bowling, 2004). A radiopaque, polyurethane tube with an internal diameter ranging from 6–12 French gauge (FG or Fr) and a minimum length of 90 centimetres is usually recommended, depending on the patient's requirements (Bowling, 2004; Best, 2005, 2007). For the purpose of gastric drainage/decompression, a larger bore polyvinyl chloride (PVC) tube is recommended (up to 22FG). However, these tubes are not advisable for feeding as they become hard and uncomfortable and can limit oral intake if the patient can eat (Bowling, 2004) (see Figure 9.1).

SYRINGES

In order to avoid incorrect administration of oral/enteral medication into the intravenous system, only specified oral/enteral feeding syringes should be used with enteral feeding systems (National Patient Safety Agency (NPSA), 2007). A purple colour has been used to differentiate these syringes from intravenous syringes (Scott, 2007)

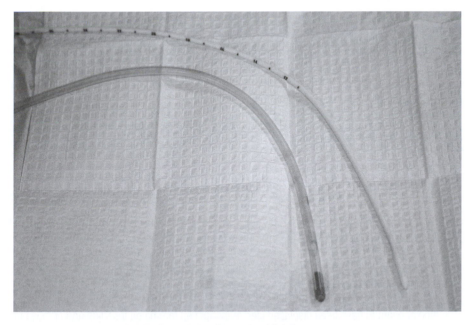

Figure 9.1   Drainage tube (left) and feeding tube (right)

PH PAPER

In order to minimise the risk of harm to patients caused by misplaced NG feeding tubes, pH indicator strips of paper should be used at the bedside when checking the gastric position of NGTs (NPSA, 2005). This requirement supersedes any previous methods used (see below).

EQUIPMENT REQUIRED

- Clinically clean tray or trolley
- Apron, non-sterile disposable gloves, protective covering for patient
- Denture pot, facial tissues, disposable receiver
- Selected nasogastric tube (adult size range from 6–12FG). Sizes may vary depending on the manufacturer
- Glass of cold water and straw. *Please note*: the patient's ability to swallow should be assessed prior to undertaking the procedure
- Catheter – tipped 50ml enteral syringes × 2
- pH indicator strips 0–6 range
- Hypoallergenic tape or securing device
- Clinical waste bag
- Fluid balance chart.

PROCEDURE – NASOGASTRIC TUBE INSERTION

Please note that this procedure is a meant as a guide; please refer to local policy and to manufacturers' instructions for all equipment used.

POINTS TO NOTE

CHECKING THE CORRECT POSITION OF THE NGT

Once the initial gastric position has been confirmed, the tube position should be checked at the following times:

- Before commencing a feed and at least once daily in continuous feeding
- Before administration of each feed
- Before administering medication
- The tube appears to have been displaced (see mark applied to tube on insertion and or loose tape)
- The patient has coughed violently, retched or vomited
- After oropharyngeal suctioning
- If the patient shows signs of respiratory distress
- When receiving a patient from another clinical area. (National Patient Safety Association (NPSA), 2005; Best, 2007)

Table 9.3

Action	Rationale	Evidence
Explain the procedure to the patient and agree a signal with the patient to stop the procedure if required	To obtain patient's consent and cooperation and give the option to withdraw from the procedure at any time	DH (2009) Best (2007)
Where possible the patient should be sitting in an upright position, supported by pillows	This position allows easy swallowing and ensures that the epiglottis is not obstructing the oesophagus	Bowling (2004)
For the semi-conscious patient, it is often easier to be in a lying position on their side	Ensures easy passage of NG tube and reduces the risk of gastric reflux	
Wash hands and apply gloves and apron (universal precautions) Assemble required equipment and select an appropriate tube	To ensure a clean procedure is maintained throughout Consider appropriate FG depending on size of the patient, diagnosis and anticipated duration of therapy Check the expiry date on packaged equipment to be used	Endacott et al. (2009) Bowling (2004)
Check nose and mouth for any signs of obstruction and ensure both are clean (after removing dentures if worn)	To aid passage of the NGT	Best (2007) Bowling (2004) Stroud et al. (2003)
Agree with the patient which nostril is to be used. You can also check nasal patency by asking patient to sniff or blow nose	Patient may have one nostril which is clearer than the other, e.g. deviated nasal septum	
Estimate the length of tube to be inserted from the tip of the nose, to the ear and xiphisternum (see Figure 9.2)	To provide an indication of when the tube reaches the stomach	Best (2007) Bowling (2004)

(Continued)

Table 9.3 (Continued)

Action	Rationale	Evidence
Flush the tube with 1–2mls of tap water Check that the guide wire moves freely	This will ensure that the guide wire can be easily removed once placed in the patient *Do not use sterile water as this has a pH of between 5 and 7*	Drugs.com (2010)
Lubricate the NG tube by immersing the end of the tube in water	This will activate the lubricant on the tip of tube (check manufacturer's instructions), facilitating easier passage when inserting the tube	Best (2007)
Insert the tube into the nostril and slide backwards and inwards along the floor of the nose to the nasopharynx approximately 10–12cm and *STOP* If any obstruction is felt, withdraw the tube slightly and try again at a slightly different angle or try the other nostril	There are two distinct stages when passing the tube: (i) Nose $\rightarrow$ pharynx $\rightarrow$ stop and swallow (ii) Pharynx $\rightarrow$ stomach	Dougherty and Lister (2008)
Ask the patient to tilt their head forward (chin to chest)	To assist the tube entering the oesophagus not the trachea	Bowling (2004)
If the patient can swallow, coincide passing the NGT with swallowing a sip of water	The passing of the NGT can be coordinated with observing for laryngeal movement. During this phase the epiglottis covers the airway and the NGT can pass into the oesophagus to elicit a swallow	Best (2007)
If the patient shows signs of respiratory distress, coughing or becomes cyanosed, remove the tube back to the nasopharynx	This may make a further attempt at tube passage more acceptable to the patient	Stroud et al. (2003)
Never advance the tube against any resistance	To prevent mucosal trauma	

Action	Rationale	Evidence
Repeat the water/swallow and advance tube to approximately 50–60cms, depending on estimated measurement	May facilitate tube advancement	
If swallow reflex is not initiated *DO NOT* continue with this method		
If you are unsuccessful, repeat the above procedure in the other nostril if tolerated by the patient. Consider a smaller bore NGT. Do not repeat procedure more than three times	One nostril may be clearer than the other. A smaller size tube may be easier to pass on specific patients	
Once at the approximate measurement, remove guide wire and secure NGT in place using securing device or hypoallergenic tape to nose and/or cheek	Most fine bore NGTs are radiopaque and do not require the guide wire to be in situ for X-ray It can also be difficult to obtain aspirate with the guide wire in situ and uncomfortable for the patient to leave the guide wire in for long periods	Best (2007)
Mark NGT with pen at point of entry into nostril	This will provide an easily identifiable mark as a baseline	
Using a 50ml enteral syringe insufflate up to 30ml of air via NGT	This clears tube of debris and forces the end of the tube away from the stomach mucosa	NPSA (2005)
Attempt to gain aspirate from NGT by *gently* withdrawing the plunger on a 50ml syringe. If aspirate is obtained, check using pH indicator strips	0.5–1ml of aspirate should be obtained The pH of aspirate should be measured using pH indicator strips in the range 1–6 with ½ point gradations	
If pH is 4 or less, you can commence feeding; usually an X-ray is not required	Indicates gastric placement	

(Continued)

Table 9.3   (Continued)

Action	Rationale	Evidence
If pH is in the range of 4–5.5, consider risk factors such as medication, i.e. proton pump inhibitors, antacids and H$_2$ antagonists before feeding	Seek advice as X-ray may be required to confirm correct gastric position	Hanna et al. (2010)
If pH 5.5 or above	*DO NOT FEED* Leave for one hour and try aspirating again If pH is still high seek advice as tube reposition or an X-ray may be required	NPSA (2005)
NB Confirmation of tube position by X-ray is only correct at the time of X-ray. Subsequent checking of position by aspirate test must be carried out at the bedside	X-ray should not be used routinely to confirm NG tube position due to risk of over exposure to radiation, cost and correct position is only verified at time of X-ray	NPSA (2005) NICE (2006)
If unable to obtain aspirate: Consider length of NGT. If measurement at nose is below approximate measure consider advancing the tube 5–10cms	Tip of tube may not be in fluid pool in the stomach – advancing the tube should enable aspirate to be obtained as tip of tube should be in gastric fluid pool	Best (2007)
If measurement at nose is above approximate measure consider withdrawing tube 5–10cms	Withdrawing tube should allow aspirate to be obtained by putting tip of tube in gastric fluid pool	NICE (2006)
Consider changing the patient's position e.g. from sitting to lying, or lying on left side	To change the fluid level in the stomach – as this may enable aspirate to be obtained	Best (2007) NICE (2006)
Inject 3–5ml of air into the tube	To push the tip away from the gastric wall	NPSA (2005)

Action	Rationale	Evidence
If still not successful, leave for one hour then try aspirating again		
If still unable to obtain aspirate and *ONLY if the patient's swallow is intact*. Encourage the patient to drink blackcurrant squash (coloured liquid) which should then be in the patient's stomach	If tip of NGT is in gastric fluid pool blackcurrant will be aspirated – *X-ray is NOT required to check position It is not safe to ask patient to drink if swallow is NOT intact*	
PTS with oesophageal stricture or oesophageal tumours will require an initial check X-ray after placement	Fluid aspirated may be from oesophagus – (not stomach) – may give a false positive ph result when tip of tube may not be in the stomach	
Following insertion and confirmation of correct position, document procedure in the patient's notes – including pH of aspirate obtained +/– confirmation by X-ray, size of tube and measurement of tube at nose	Accountability for checking the tube position before use lies with the competent healthcare professional Recording the procedure is a requirement in law and provides a baseline for further measurement *NB: This is a legal requirement*	NMC (2005)

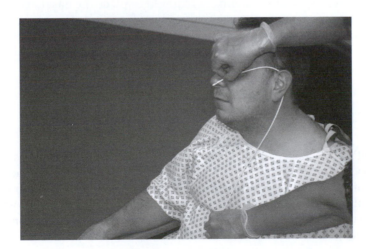

Figure 9.2

It is important that the pH aspirate is measured using pH indicator strips/paper as other methods such as using blue litmus paper, auscultation of air syringed into the NGT, observing the appearance of the aspirate only, immersion of the hub of the tube in water and inspecting for bubbles, interpretation of absence of respiratory distress or impaired phonation are not reliable and could lead to misinterpretation of the tube position (NPSA, 2005).

FEEDING POSITION

If a patient is bed bound, on overnight feeding and/or has dysphagia, they should be positioned at 30–45° at least during feeding and for 45–60 minutes afterwards (Bowling, 2004; Best, 2005).

FIXATION DEVICES

NGTs have traditionally been secured to the nose and/or cheek using adhesive, hypoallergenic tape. Unfortunately, while NGTs are relatively easy to place, they can also easily be dislodged by restless or cognitively impaired patients (Williams, 2005). Furthermore, tape does not adhere well to skin for prolonged periods of time due to moisture, grease and nasal secretions accumulating on the skin.

An alternative to adhesive tape is the nasal bridle or loop where there is an increased risk of displacement, e.g. in dysphagic stroke patients (Horsburgh et al., 2008). The placement of this device involves the passage of a length of cotton tape behind the nasal septum which is then secured to the NGT and is useful to maintain enteral access while decisions are made with regard to long-term feeding. However, specialist training is required to place the nasal bridle and there are ethical issues, particularly weighing up benefits versus harm, e.g. discomfort and trauma in patients with severe cognitive impairment such as those with a head injury or advanced dementia (Williams, 2005; Best, 2007; Horsburgh et al., 2008).

BODY IMAGE

The patient's body image should also be taken into consideration as NGTs and fixation devices can be perceived as unsightly and an outward sign of ill health. Therefore, if enteral tube feeding is required long term, that is, for more than four weeks, an alternative route of feeding should be considered, e.g. gastrostomy feeding or jejunal feeding in patients with upper gastrointestinal dysfunction or an inaccessible upper gastrointestinal tract (NICE, 2006).

TUBE PATENCY

Inadequate flushing is the most common cause of tube blockage (British Association Parental and Enteral Nutrition (BAPEN), 2004). Therefore NGTs should be flushed with at least 30ml water and using a 50ml enteral syringe before and after feed and drug administration (Bowling, 2004; Roberts, 2007).

DRUG ADMINISTRATION

Medication administered via feeding tubes and where its original preparation has been changed, e.g. by crushing a tablet, generally falls outside the drug product licence (BAPEN, 2004). Therefore, to minimise the risk of any possible complications, a pharmacist should be consulted with regard to the most appropriate drug preparation to use (Best, 2005).

Using the wrong drug preparation is also a common cause of tube blockage (BAPEN, 2004). Therefore the tube should be flushed with at least 30ml of water before drug administration via a tube, with at least 10ml in between drugs if more than one drug is used, and with at least 30ml after the last drug (BAPEN, 2004). A step-by-step guide can be accessed on http://www.bapen.org.uk/res_drugs.html (BAPEN, 2004).

ADMINISTRATION OF FEED

The enteral feed to be delivered via the NG tube comes in a variety of different formulations which vary in relation to energy, protein, fat, fibre, fluid and micronutrient content (NICE, 2006). The feed will usually be prescribed by a dietician following a thorough nutritional assessment and calculation of the patient's nutritional requirements. The ETF is then delivered through a giving set and via a pump over a set period of time within 24 hours depending on the patient's clinical circumstances and the feed to be delivered, 16–18 hours is usually sufficient (Bowling, 2004; Roberts, 2007). Bolus feeding, that is, administration of feed via an enteral syringe, is an alternative method of feed administration in some patients (Roberts, 2007).

The expiry date and packaging of enteral feeding equipment should be checked before use, that is, giving sets and bags of feed, and routinely changed after 24 hours to minimise the risk of bacterial contamination (Best, 2005).

MAINTAINING HYDRATION AND NUTRITION

An accurate record of fluid balance should be maintained and fluid balance monitored closely as there may be a risk of fluid and electrolyte imbalance, particularly if a patient has undergone a period of fasting prior to starting NG feeding (Stroud et al., 2003; NICE, 2006).

If vomiting, diarrhoea or abdominal bloating occurs the feed rate should be slowed or stopped depending on severity, and reported to the dietician and medical team to review cause and hydration status.

The patient should undergo nutritional screening at least weekly and according to local policy (NICE, 2006).

Insertion of a Fine Bore Enteral Feeding Tube

Aim

For learners safely to pass a fine bore feeding tube and understand the importance of monitoring for potential complications associated with tube insertion and maintenance of hydration and nutrition.

Objectives

By the end of this scenario the learner should be able to:

- Demonstrate a knowledge of normal anatomy, physiology of upper gastrointestinal, respiratory tract and the physiology of swallowing
- Discuss the indications and contraindications of enteral tube feeding
- Identify the range of NGTs and select the appropriate enteral tube for feeding
- Gather appropriate equipment and prepare the patient for the procedure, including obtaining informed consent
- Demonstrate the correct procedure for estimating the length of NGT to be inserted
- Safely pass the NGT, secure into place and check that it is correctly positioned in the stomach
- Identify reasons for failing to gain gastric aspirate and how to remedy this
- Explain what information needs documenting in the nursing/medical records
- Discuss the monitoring and prevention of potential complications of NG feeding
- Discuss the importance of nutrition and maintaining a fluid balance chart.

Resources

Equipment

- Clinically clean tray or trolley
- Apron, non-sterile disposable gloves, protective covering for patient
- Denture pot, facial tissues, disposable receiver
- Selected nasogastric tube (adult size range from 6–12FG); sizes may vary depending on the manufacturer
- Glass of cold water and a straw. NB: The patient's ability to swallow should be assessed prior to undertaking the procedure
- 50ml enteral/catheter tipped syringe × 2
- pH indicator strips 0–6 range

- Hypoallergenic tape or securing device
- Clinical waste bag
- Fluid balance chart.

Time Element

See Table 9.4 (timings are approximate).

Table 9.4

Process	Time Element
Introduction, aims and objectives of session	10 minutes
Recap normal upper gastrointestinal/respiratory anatomy and physiology including the physiology of swallowing	15 minutes
Identify different types of NGTs and discuss the indications/contraindications	15 minutes
Preparation of equipment	5 minutes
Preparation of patient/manikin including explanation of procedure, gaining informed consent and correct position	15 minutes
Insertion of NGT, correct procedure for checking tube position and securing tube	30 minutes
Discuss the procedures to follow if no gastric aspirate obtained	10 minutes
Documentation in patient's records and completing fluid balance chart	5 minutes
Discuss the reasons when the NGT position needs checking	10 minutes
Conclusion/summary to session Discussion points	30 minutes

Settings

- Hospital ward at patient's bedside
- Clinical skills suite/practical room.

Roles of Participants

Facilitator

- To lead discussion with the learner group
- To demonstrate the procedure to the learners then act as supervisor as the learner practises the procedure.

Learners

- One learner to undertake the procedure under the supervision of the facilitator
- To participate in discussions.

Other members of group should participate in observing and giving feedback to the learner.

Areas for Discussion

- Patient consent
- NGT position check
- Drug administration via NGT
- Fixation techniques
- Psychological impact of NGT
- Monitoring of nutritional status
- Effects of malnutrition on patient outcomes.

REFERENCES

Best, C. (2005) 'Caring for the patient with a nasogastric tube', *Nursing Standard*, 20 (3): 59–65.

Best, C. (2007) 'Nasogastric tube insertion in adults who require enteral feeding', *Nursing Standard*, 21 (40): 39–43.

Bowling, T. (ed.) (2004) *Nutritional Support for Adults and Children. A Handbook for Hospital Practice*. Oxford: Radcliffe Medical Press.

British Association of Parental and Enteral Nutrition (BAPEN) (2004) *Administering Drugs via Enteral Feeding Tubes: A Practical Guide*. Available on: http://www.bapen.org.uk/res_drugs.html [accessed on 8 February 2011].

British Association of Parental and Enteral Nutrition (BAPEN) (2009) *£13 Billion Cost of Malnutrition Must be Tackled*. Media release, available on: http://www.bapen.org.uk/pdfs/press_releases/press_42.pdf [accessed 1 October 2010].

British Medical Association (2007) *Withholding and Withdrawing Life-prolonging Medical Treatment: Guidance for Decision Making*, 3rd edn. Oxford: Blackwell Publishing.

Colbert, B., Ankey, J., Lee, K., Steggall, M. and Dingle, M. (2009) *Anatomy and Physiology for Nursing and Health Professionals*. Essex: Pearson Education.

Department of Health (DH) (2009) *Reference Guide to Consent for Examination or Treatment*, 2nd edn. Available on: http://webarchive.nationalarchives.gov.uk/+/www.dh.gov.uk/en/Publichealth/Scientificdevelopmentgeneticsandbioethics/Consent/index.htm [accessed 9 February 2011].

Dougherty, L. and Lister, S. (eds) (2008) *The Royal Marsden Hospital Manual of Clinical Nursing Procedures*, Student Edition, 7th edn. Oxford: Wiley-Blackwell.

Drugs.com (2010) Drug Information Online. Available on: http://www.drugs.com/pro/sterile-water-for-injection.html [accessed 8 February 2011].

Endacott, R., Jevon, P. and Cooper, S. (2009) *Clinical Nursing Skills Core and Advanced*. Oxford: Oxford University Press.

Hanna, G., Phillips, L., Prielst, O. and Ni, Z. (2010) *Improving the Safety of Nasogastric Feeding Tube Insertion. A Report for the NHS Patient Safety Research Portfolio*. Available on: http://www.haps.bham.ac.uk/publichealth/psrp/documents/PS048_Improving_the_safety_of_nasogastric_feeding_tube_insertion_REVISED_Hanna_et_al.pdf [accessed 2 February 2011].

Horsburgh, D., Rowat, A. and Mahoney, C. (2008) 'A necessary evil? Interventions to prevent nasogastric tube-tugging after stroke', *British Journal of Neuroscience*, 4 (5): 230–4.

Malnutrition Advisory Group (2003) 'A consistent and reliable tool for malnutrition screening', *Nursing Times*, 99 (46): 26–7.

May, S. (2007) 'Testing nasogastric tube positioning in the critically ill: exploring the evidence', *British Journal of Nursing*, 16 (7): 414–18.

Mental Capacity Act (2005) Available on: http://webarchive.nationalarchives.gov.uk/*/http://www.dca.gov.uk/ [accessed 9 February 2011].

National Institute for Clinical Excellence (NICE) (2006) *Nutrition Support in Adults. Oral Nutrition Support, Enteral Tube Feeding and Parenteral Nutrition*. London: National Collaborating Centre for Acute Care.

National Patient Safety Agency (NPSA) (2005) *Reducing the Harm Caused by Misplaced Nasogastric Feeding Tubes. How to Confirm the Correct Position of Nasogastric Feeding Tubes in Infants, Children and Adults*. London: NPSA. Available on: http://www.nrls.npsa.nhs.uk/resources/?EntryId45=59794 [accessed 9 February 2011].

National Patient Safety Agency (NPSA) (2007) *Patient Safety Alert. Promoting Safer Measurement and Administration of Liquid Medicines via Oral and other Enteral Routes*. Ref NPSA/2007/19. Available on: http://www.nrls.npsa.nhs.uk/resources/?entryid45=59808 [accessed 9 February 2011].

Nursing and Midwifery Council (NMC) (2005) *Guidelines for Records and Record Keeping*. London: NMC.

Nursing and Midwifery Council (NMC) (2008) *The Code: Standards of Conduct, Performance and Ethics for Nurses and Midwives*. London: NMC.

Roberts, E. (2007) 'Nutritional support via enteral tube feeding in hospital patients', *British Journal of Nursing*, 16 (17): 1058–62.

Royal College of Physicians (RCP) (2010) *Oral Feeding Difficulties and Dilemmas. A Guide to Practical Care, Particularly Towards the End of Life*. London: Royal College of Physicians.

Scott, S. (2007) 'Quick compliance with safety alert on oral/enteral syringes. Policy and practice: patient safety', *Hospital Pharmacy Europe*. Available on: www.baxa.com [accessed 9 February 2011].

Stroud, M., Duncan, H. and Nightingale, J. (2003) 'Guidelines for enteral feeding in adult hospital patients', *GUT*, 52 (suppl 7): vii1 – vii12. Available on: http://www.bsg.org.uk/images/stories/docs/clinical/guidelines/sbn/enteral.pdf [accessed 9 February 2011].

Williams, J. (2005) 'Using an alternative fixing device for nasogastric tubes', *Nursing Times*, 101 (35): 26–7.

10

INFECTION PREVENTION: ASEPTIC NON-TOUCH TECHNIQUE, HAND WASHING, DISPOSAL OF SHARPS AND DISPOSAL OF WASTE

Mandy Reynolds

Aim

The aim of this chapter is to give ideas and scenarios to facilitate the teaching of four key areas of infection prevention and control: aseptic technique, hand hygiene, sharps disposal and waste disposal.

Objectives

At the end of this chapter the reader will be able to:

- Discuss the importance of appropriate infection prevention practice in healthcare settings
- Identify how infections are transmitted and how this can be prevented
- Describe techniques to facilitate learning which will, in turn, develop a knowledge base and skills to encourage good infection prevention practice in the clinical area.

INTRODUCTION TO THE SKILL

Infection prevention and control education is integral to the continuing education of healthcare workers (Billings, 2010). Healthcare associated infection (HCAI) has become a high-profile problem in recent years, with regular attention from the media. It is a serious concern which causes approximately 5000 deaths per year and costs the National Health Service (NHS) £1 billion pounds per year (Aziz, 2009).

Although HCAIs are not a new problem, the type of infections seen in healthcare establishments have changed; for example, in the 1800s HCAI included typhus, dysentery and scabies. In more modern times we see, for example, *Methicillin-Resistant Staphylococcus Aureus* (MRSA) and *Clostridium Difficile* (Gould and Brooker, 2000). There are also new emerging 'super bugs', for example Extended spectrum B-Lactamases.

BACKGROUND TO THE SKILL

The management and control of HCAIs has been a matter of priority for the NHS for a number of years (Downie et al., 2010). The current phase of the Department of Health (DH) strategy for HCAI is clearly outlined in the publication *Clean, Safe Care* (DH, 2008). It states that the focus of attention is on healthcare providers who need to demonstrate, year on year, a reduction in all avoidable HCAI to the 'irreducible minimum' (Robertson, 2009). The Health and Social Care Act 2008 Code of Practice (DH, 2009) states that it is the responsibility of every healthcare worker to help reduce HCAIs and that effective prevention and control of HCAIs has to be applied consistently by everyone. A reduction has been seen in HCAIs in healthcare establishments, but there are still preventable deaths every year due to patients contracting an HCAI.

There is evidence to suggest that knowledge of and compliance with infection prevention protocols among healthcare workers is very poor (Reime et al., 2008). It has been shown that suboptimal practice of healthcare workers is the main cause of HCAI transmission (Wilson, 2007) through, for example, poor hand hygiene and aseptic techniques. Infection prevention and control education is integral to the induction and continuing education of all healthcare professionals (Billings, 2010).

TRANSMISSION OF PATHOGENS

The different stages by which transient pathogens succeed in causing infection are collectively called the chain of infection. This has to be broken in order to prevent the spread of infections (Ayling, 2007).

This chain can be summarised as follows:

- The chain of infection begins with a living pathogen being present in the environment
- The pathogen then needs a route of transmission, for example, hands or food
- It then requires a port of entry into the host, for example, mouth or broken skin
- Once in the body the pathogen will multiply, causing the host to feel unwell
- Pathogens leave the host via an exit route to contaminate the environment.

INTRODUCTION TO ASEPTIC NON-TOUCH TECHNIQUE (ANTT)

Poor aseptic technique has been shown to be a major cause of HCAI (The Association of Safe Aseptic Practice (ASAP), 2011). ANTT was introduced by the DH in 2006 in an effort to provide a framework to reduce HCAI (Lewis, 2009). It is a standardised approach to aseptic practice which has been shown to reduce HCAIs significantly (Rowley and Clare, 2009; ASAP, 2011). The educator can demonstrate any aseptic procedure that is applicable to the audience, for example, wound care, urinary catheterisation, suturing or inserting venous cannulas. This scenario can be carried out as a one-to-one or group session.

LEARNING OBJECTIVES

The objectives of this simulation are to:

- Demonstrate, practise and discuss the procedure
- Enable the practitioner to perform the skill and understand the principles of ANTT in order to minimise the risk of introducing microorganisms into a vulnerable site.

RESOURCES

EQUIPMENT

Table 10.1

Equipment	Rationale
Metal aseptic trolley	Easily decontaminated to prevent cross infection
Alcohol disinfectant	To decontaminate the trolley before the procedure
Sterile packs and other equipment needed	
Gloves	To protect the healthcare professional from bodily fluids
Apron	To protect the healthcare professional's clothing from splash contamination
Sharps box (if required)	To dispose of sharps at point of use
Waste bin/bag	To dispose of clinical waste at point of use
Hand wash sink	To decontaminate hands before the procedure
Hand soap	To decontaminate hands before the procedure
Hand gel	To decontaminate hands at key points during the procedure
Manikin limb	In place of a patient

SETTING

This scenario could take place in either a clinical setting or in a classroom, providing there is access to a hand wash sink.

TIME ELEMENT

It will take approximately 15 minutes to explain the procedure and a further 15 minutes to observe the practice of each participant.

PROCEDURE

Table 10.2

Action	Rationale
Hands to be washed with soap and water	To be decontaminated before procedure
Collect the aseptic trolley and clean with an alcohol-based disinfectant. Start with spraying the cleaning fluid all over the trolley. Ideally this should be left to dry but if time is of the essence the trolley can be dabbed dry – using clean paper towels, from the back of the trolley to the front and from the top to the wheels	To decontaminate the trolley before the procedure to avoid cross contamination from the trolley to the sterile packs and hands
Decontaminate hands with soap and water or gel	To remove any microbes that could have been transferred from the dirty trolley to hands
Collect all the equipment needed to perform the task and place on the bottom shelf of the trolley. Check all packaging for damage and the use-by dates on collection	To have all equipment to hand; this will in turn help to avoid contamination due to unnecessary movement
Proceed to the area where the task is to be completed. Explain the procedure to the patient and ensure that they are comfortable	To ensure that it is the correct patient and that they are fully informed to enable consent for the procedure
Proceed to open the sterile packs starting with the pack that will become the sterile field. Ensure the contents are not touched when being opened and that the outer packaging does not touch the top shelf of the trolley (see Figure 10.1)	To avoid contamination of the sterile field

(Continued)

Table 10.2   (Continued)

Action	Rationale
Decontaminate hands before spreading the pack out. Handle as little as possible, only touching the corners	Hands are to be decontaminated at this point to avoid contamination of sterile pack from any microbes that could have been picked up on the hands from the outer packaging
The objects in the pack can be spread on the sterile field by inserting a hand into the sterile waste bag included in the pack. The bag can also be used to remove the dressing if present. Attach the bag to the trolley, nearest side to the patient	Using the bag will avoid any unnecessary handling of the equipment and reduce contamination of hands when removing the dressing
The rest of the sterile equipment can now be emptied onto the sterile field. Open the packs as before without the outer packaging touching the sterile field or hands touching the contents. The non-sterile equipment should be kept on the bottom shelf until needed	To prevent contamination of equipment
Decontaminate hands before proceeding to move the sterile towel to the patient so there is a second sterile field. Again handle the towel as little as possible by only touching the corners	To avoid contamination from hands, as microbes could have been picked up from the outer packaging
Apply gloves and proceed with the procedure. At this point the participant should be aware that they have a 'clean' and 'dirty' hand. The 'dirty' hand should be used to carry out the task with only the 'clean' hand touching the objects on the sterile field. The objects are to be transferred from the 'clean' hand to the dirty' hand without hands touching and away from the sterile field	The 'clean' and 'dirty' hand method is used to ensure that the sterile field is not contaminated with any microbes from the patient
The clinical waste should be deposited in the appropriate waste bag as per local policy and sharps should be disposed of appropriately at the point of use	To ensure safe disposal of waste
Apron to be removed and trolley cleaned with detergent wipes	To ensure the trolley is left clean after the procedure
Procedure to be documented in the patient's notes as per local policy	To enable good practice of documentation and to inform others of the procedure having been carried out

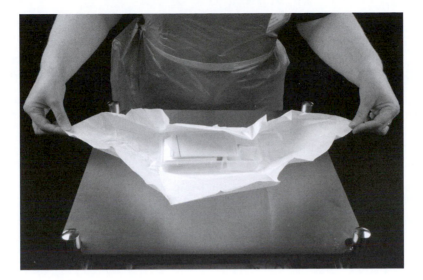

Figure 10.1

DISCUSSION

The skill should be demonstrated by the assessor in the first instance and then the practitioner should be assessed. It should be made clear that the practitioner is being assessed only on their ANTT and not on the task being carried out, for example, the insertion of a peripheral venous cannula.

The rationale for each step needs to be explained to ensure that the participant understands the reason for using this technique.

HAND HYGIENE

INTRODUCTION TO HAND HYGIENE

Hand hygiene in the clinical setting has been discussed since the 1800s. It is the quickest and easiest way to help prevent the spread of HCAIs but it is disappointing that many healthcare professionals do not appreciate its importance. Adherence rates to hand hygiene protocols are frequently reported to be less than 50% (Ruef, 2009). Some of the reasons for non-compliance with hand hygiene include skin irritation, forgetting, and the belief that the use of gloves negates the need for decontaminating hands (Torner, 2009).

Hands can be contaminated with microorganisms not only from contact with a patient but also from equipment or the patient's environment (Wilson, 2007).

One of the first healthcare professionals to research the effect of hand hygiene was Ignaz Semmelweis in 1800. He carried out an audit on the effect of hand washing by doctors on wound infections and found that it reduced the amount of infections in wounds (Lane et al., 2010). More recently the following guidance has been given by the World Health Organization (WHO) on correct handwashing technique in the clinical setting (see Figure 10.2) (WHO, 2009).

The WHO also identify the five moments for hand hygiene which are:

- Before an aseptic task
- Before patient contact
- After patient contact
- After contact with the patient's surroundings
- After contact with bodily fluids.

How to Handwash?

WASH HANDS WHEN VISIBLY SOILED! OTHERWISE, USE HANDRUB

🕐 **Duration of the entire procedure:** 40-60 seconds

0 Wet hands with water;

1 Apply enough soap to cover all hand surfaces;

2 Rub hands palm to palm;

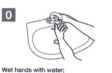

3 Right palm over left dorsum with interlaced fingers and vice versa;

4 Palm to palm with fingers interlaced;

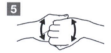

5 Backs of fingers to opposing palms with fingers interlocked;

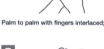

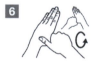

6 Rotational rubbing of left thumb clasped in right palm and vice versa;

7 Rotational rubbing, backwards and forwards with clasped fingers of right hand in left palm and vice versa;

8 Rinse hands with water;

9 Dry hands thoroughly with a single use towel;

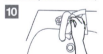

10 Use towel to turn off faucet;

11 Your hands are now safe.

World Health Organization | **Patient Safety** A World Alliance for Safer Health Care | **SAVE LIVES** Clean **Your** Hands

May 2009

Figure 10.2

Source: World Health Organization (2009) *How to Handwash*. Available at: www.who.int/gpsc/5may/How_To_HandWash_Poster.pdf

It is not just the times at which hand decontamination takes place that is important but also the technique that is used. The tips of fingers, palms of hands, wrists and finger-web spaces are typically missed when carrying out hand hygiene, therefore, they can still be covered in microorganisms (Ayling, 2007). A good hand-washing technique is essential to ensure that all areas of the hand and wrist are included when carrying out hand decontamination. It is also important that the healthcare professional is bare below the elbow in the clinical area to ensure that the whole of the hand and wrist can be decontaminated (DH, 2007).

INTRODUCTION TO THE SCENARIO

Role-play can be effective in demonstrating the principles of hand hygiene. Acting out clinical situations and having the audience decide if hand hygiene is appropriate at certain times can help make the practitioner think more deeply about their own practice and how it can be improved.

LEARNING OBJECTIVES

The practitioner will become aware of the importance of performing effective hand hygiene

- The practitioner will understand the principles of the WHO five moments for hand hygiene in the clinical setting
- The practitioner will understand the principles requiring them to be bare below the elbow.

RESOURCES

EQUIPMENT

Table 10.3

Equipment	Rationale
'Role players'	They would be needed to act out scenes as patients and staff
Clinical equipment	Such as blood pressure recording machines, notes trolley, drug trolley, aseptic trolley, sharps trays, etc.
Hand wash sink	To demonstrate hand washing
Hand gel	As an alternative to hand washing
Pre-planned scenarios	See below
Hand hygiene audit	To enable good and bad practice to be recorded for discussion

SETTING

This scenario could be carried out in the clinical setting or in a clinical resource room. If neither of these is available, then a classroom could be used with signs to represent the presence of a hand wash sink, etc.

TIME ELEMENT

This scenario would take at least 60 minutes to give time for the explanation of the WHO five moments for hand hygiene, the hand hygiene audit and the scenario; this would also include the run through the role-play and the results at the end of the session.

SIMULATION SCENARIO

Scenario – Procedure

Table 10.4

Action	Rationale
The actors would demonstrate tasks, for example, taking the blood pressure of a patient then going to another patient to take a temperature, or straightening the bed clothes of a patient before performing an aseptic technique	Any tasks can be used to demonstrate work carried out in a clinical area
The 'role players' would demonstrate appropriate hand hygiene, or not, between tasks	This would give the audience the opportunity to document whether appropriate hand hygiene was carried out
Several opportunities would be given for hand hygiene between different tasks. These can be done at the same time to make it more challenging or one after the other	It may make the scene more interesting if a couple of actions are being played out at the same time. If the audience is finding it difficult, then it can be scaled down to one action at a time
The audience would document on their hand hygiene audit whether hand hygiene was performed at the appropriate times	As the audience will be using the same format to document the actions, it will be easier to discuss at the end
A discussion would then take place to determine when the opportunities for hand hygiene took place and whether they were acted upon accurately	The tasks and audience opinions can be discussed, therefore, promoting good practice

Discussion

The audience will need background knowledge of hand hygiene to be able to recognise whether effective hand hygiene is being performed at the appropriate times. Effective hand hygiene would not be documented on the hand hygiene audit but this can be raised as part of the discussion at the end.

SHARPS DISPOSAL

INTRODUCTION TO SHARPS DISPOSAL

Throughout this chapter the term 'sharps' refers to any sharp instrument or equipment, for example, needles and blades. Needle stick injuries are a hazard for all healthcare workers with not only a risk of transmission of blood-borne viruses such as Hepatitis B, Hepatitis C and Human Immunodeficiency Virus (HIV) but also psychological injury. An irresponsible attitude towards sharps disposal is not uncommon among healthcare professionals, putting other healthcare workers at risk (Blenkharn, 2009).

Although it is usually believed that front line healthcare workers are most at risk of a sharps injury, a study in the United States shows that support staff are 10 times more likely to sustain an injury than nurses, and 30 to 40 times more likely than medical staff (Leigh et al., 2008). This is due to needles and other sharp instruments being placed in inappropriate clinical waste receptacles (Blenkharn, 2009).

It has been found that the majority of injuries that take place in the clinical area are between the point of use and disposal of the sharps (Scottish Executive, 2001). Recommendations from research into needle stick injuries state that sharps containers should be taken to the point of use to help minimise this risk of injury (Pratt et al., 2007).

The Scottish Executive (2001) advises that the following principles should be used when handling sharps:

- Use needleless devices whenever possible
- Do not re-sheath needles
- Never pass sharps from person to person by hand
- Never walk around with a sharp
- Always dispose of sharps yourself at the point of use
- Dispose of needles and syringes as a single unit
- Remove the needle and attach a blind hub to a blood gas syringe when transporting (Scottish Executive, 2001)
- Never overfill the sharps bin
- Ensure the lid is closed when the sharps bin is not in use
- Always use standard precautions.

Other points to be considered include:

- Always ensure sharps containers are assembled and labelled properly
- Never carry a sharps container close to the body but use the handle or tray
- Sharps containers should be locked before disposal and stored in a locked cupboard while awaiting collection.

LEARNING OBJECTIVES

- The principles of safe disposal of sharps will be discussed
- The practitioner will be encouraged to think about their own practice and how it can be improved in the clinical setting.

RESOURCES

EQUIPMENT

Table 10.5

Equipment	Rationale
Role players	To act as healthcare professionals and demonstrate good and poor practice of sharps disposal To act as patients
Side room or clinical skills room	Provides an appropriate venue
Sharps containers and trays	To dispose of sharps at point of use
Different types/items of sharps, for example, needles and syringes, blades, etc.	For demonstration purposes
Personal protective equipment	To demonstrate best practice
Hand decontamination facilities	To demonstrate appropriate hand hygiene
Video camera	To record the scenes on tape

SETTING

The skills would be demonstrations of care given at a patient's bedside, in a theatre, or in an outpatients' clinic.

TIME ELEMENT

The time to be taken on this session would depend on the number of video clips shown and the length of the discussion which follows the session. The scenes should be kept short to encourage audience discussion and interaction (Billings, 2010).

Scenario – Procedure

Table 10.6

Action	Rationale
The following scenario would be filmed	Scenarios would then be available to be viewed when needed
A room would be set up as a clinical area with role players as healthcare professionals and patients	To demonstrate the care being given in a clinical setting
The healthcare professional would approach the patient to give an intra-muscular injection carrying a sharps box and a needle and syringe	To demonstrate good practice of sharps disposal at the point of use
The healthcare professional would explain the procedure to the patient and check their ID while decontaminating their hands with hand gel	Hand decontamination is needed at this point as they are going to be in contact with the patient
The patient would be prepared and the injection given	
The needle and syringe would be deposited into the sharps box at the point of use, the lid of the box would be closed and the patient made comfortable	Demonstrating disposal of sharps at the point of use and closing the lid of the sharps box to avoid sharps injuries
The healthcare professional would gel their hands before leaving the patient's environment	Demonstrating good hand hygiene in the clinical area
The sharps tray and box would be cleaned with a detergent wipe	To demonstrate good infection control practice after the equipment has been brought out of a patient's environment

SIMULATION SCENARIO

Discussion

The procedure outlined above is one example of a scene that could be filmed. Several different scenarios could be filmed of good and poor practice, again to be discussed at the end. The audience would need some background knowledge of the regulations regarding the disposal of sharps.

Consideration would need to be given to the safety of participants when acting out the scenes to avoid injury. The scenes could be filmed to avoid using actual sharps, but if they do need to be demonstrated then only clean sharps are to be used. Sharps disposal would be the main focus of these scenarios but other infection control practices would need to be demonstrated appropriately, such as hand decontamination.

WASTE DISPOSAL

INTRODUCTION TO WASTE DISPOSAL

It is every healthcare worker's responsibility to dispose of waste appropriately and safely. If procedures for carrying out waste disposal are not observed, other infection prevention procedures that you perform could be undermined (Ayling, 2007). There are different types of waste found in clinical settings. These include household, clinical and biological waste. The term 'clinical waste' refers to any bodily fluid, wound dressings, contaminated pads, aprons, gloves and small plastic instruments. Biological waste is any fluid that has the potential to contaminate objects, damage skin or affect breathing. There is guidance and legislation behind the segregation and disposal of waste. The Environmental Protection (Duty of Care) Regulations (1991) state that all producers of waste must take responsibility for ensuring that their waste is disposed of without harm to human health or the environment.

The Health and Social Care Act (DH, 2008) also advises that the precautions listed below be included in connection with the handling of healthcare waste:

- Training and information
- Segregation of wastes
- The use of appropriate PPE
- Immunisation
- Appropriate procedures for handling waste
- Appropriate packaging and labelling
- Suitable transport
- A clear procedure for dealing with accidents and spills
- Appropriate treatment and disposal of waste.

This scenario encourages the practitioner to think about what kind of waste is being discarded and whether it is going into the appropriate receptacle.

RESOURCES

EQUIPMENT

Table 10.7

Equipment	Rationale
Clinical and non-clinical waste, for example: • incontinence pads • newspapers • intravenous line • tissues • dressings	For examples of waste found in a clinical area
Different types of waste bags, depending on what is available locally	To dispose of the waste
Personal protective equipment: • Aprons • Gloves • Masks • Eye protection	To protect from bodily fluids and splash injuries
Hand gel/soap and water	To decontaminate hands

SETTING

This scenario can be carried out in a side room, clinical resource room or a classroom. The room would be set up as if a patient had been discharged. If a classroom is used, a little more imagination is needed. The clinical and non-clinical waste would be left around the room, for example, the incontinence pad which has been wet with water would be left on the bed. Tissues and cordial bottle would be left on the locker. An intravenous infusion set would be left on a drip stand.

Scenario

Table 10.8

Action	Rationale
A room to be prepared as if a patient had been discharged. Several items of waste to be left in the room as above	To demonstrate the type of waste left when a patient is discharged
Participants to be given a waste bag and an example from each waste stream	To inform the participants of the types of existing waste streams
Participants to enter the room and collect the waste appropriate for their waste bags	To encourage thought as to which waste is appropriate for which waste stream and to encourage discussion
Observe the way the bag is closed	The swan neck knot is the safest to ensure spills do not occur
Ask where the waste bag would be kept while awaiting collection from the clinical area	To ensure the correct procedure is known
Once all the waste is collected, a discussion could be encouraged around whether the waste in the bags is appropriate for that particular waste stream bag	To encourage discussion on the different waste collected

Time Element

Time would need to be set aside for the setting up of the room and for collecting all the equipment needed for this scenario.

The scenario itself would take as long as would be needed for the participants to make a decision as to how each item of waste was to be discarded. Time will also need to be allocated at the end for a discussion/debrief.

Discussion

This scenario will encourage discussion and debate into waste disposal. Local waste regulations can be discussed during the scenario or at the debrief at the end. The continuing journey of the waste once it has left the clinical area could be discussed to encourage better understanding of the reasons for segregating waste.

REFERENCES

Association of Safe Aseptic Practice (ASAP) (2011) *Why Use ANTT?* Available on: http:// wwww.ant.org.uk/antt_site/care-guidelines.html [accessed 11 January 2011].

Ayling, P. (2007) *Infection Prevention and Control.* Oxford: Harcourt Education Ltd.

Aziz, A. (2009) 'Variations in aseptic technique and implications for infection control', *British Journal of Nursing,* 18 (1): 26–31.

Billings, A. (2010) 'Lights, camera, infection prevention action', *Journal of Infection Prevention,* 11 (6): 222–7.

Blenkharn, J.I. (2009) 'Sharps management and the disposal of clinical waste', *British Journal of Nursing,* 18 (14): 860–4.

Department of Environment, Food and Rural Affairs (1990) *Environmental Protection Act, Waste Management, The Duty of Care, A Code of Practice.* Available on: http://archive. defra.gov.uk/environment/waste/controls/documents/waste-man-duty-code.pdf [accessed 11 November 2011].

Department of Health (2007) *Uniforms and Workwear: an Evidence Base for Developing Local Policy.* Available on: http://www.dh.gov.uk/publications [accessed 14 March 2011].

Department of Health (2008) *Clean, Safe Care: Reducing Infection and Saving Lives.* London: HMSO.

Department of Health (2009) *The Health and Social Care Act 2008: Code of Practice for the NHS on the Prevention and Control of Healthcare Associated Infections and Related Guidance.* London: The Stationery Office.

Downie, F., Egdell, S., Bielby, A. and Searle, R. (2010) 'Barrier dressings in surgical site infection prevention strategies', *British Journal of Nursing,* 19 (20): S42–S46.

Gould, D. and Brooker, C. (2000) *Applied Microbiology for Nurses.* Basingstoke: Palgrave Macmillan.

Lane, H.J., Blum, N. and Fee, H. (2010) 'Oliver Wendell Holmes (1809–1894) and Ignaz Philipp Semmelweis (1818–1865): preventing the transmission of puerperal fever', *American Journal of Public Health,* 100 (6): 1008–9.

Leigh, J.P.O., Waitrowski, W.J., Gillen, M. and Steenland, N.K. (2008) 'Characteristics of persons and jobs with needlestick injuries in a national data set', *American Journal of Infection Control,* 36 (6): 414–20.

Lewis, G. (2009) 'ANTT clinical competencies for nursing students', *Australian Nursing Journal,* 17 (4): 39–41.

Pratt, R.J., Pellowe, C.M., Wilson, J.A., Loveday, H.P., Harper, P.J., Jones, S.R.L.J., McDougall, C. and Wilcox, M.H. (2007) 'Epic 2: national evidence-based guidelines for preventing healthcare-associated infections in NHS hospitals in England', *Journal of Hospital Infection,* 65 (1): S1–S65.

Reime, M.H., Harris, A., Aksnes, J. and Mikkelsen, J. (2008) 'The most successful method in teaching nursing students infection control – E learning or lecture?', *Nurse Education Today,* 28 (7): 798–806.

Robertson, Y. (2009) 'Root cause analysis for HCAI'. Available on: http://www.ips.uknet/ admin/uploads/conference%20presentations/north%20east/root_cause_analysis [accessed 19 January 2011].

Rowley, S. and Clare, S. (2009) 'Improving standards of aseptic practice through ANTT trust-wide implementation process: a matter of prioritisation and care', *Journal of Infection Prevention,* 10 (1): 18–23.

Ruef, C. (2009) 'Hand hygiene: adherence influenced by knowledge and subjective norms', *Infection*, 37 (4): 295.

Scottish Executive (2001) *Needlestick Injuries: Sharpen Your Awareness. Report on the Short Life Working Group on Needlestick Injuries in the NHS Scotland.* Edinburgh: Scottish Executive.

Torner, N. (2009) 'Hand hygiene focus yields visible results', *Materials Management in Health Care,* November, 2009.

Wilson, J. (2007) *Infection Control in Clinical Practice,* 3rd edn. London: BailliereTindall.

World Health Organization (WHO) (2009) *WHO Guidelines on Hand Hygiene in Healthcare. First Global Patient Safety Challenge: Clean Care is Safer Care.* Available on: http://whqlibdoc.who.int/publications/20099789241597906_eng.pdf [accessed 22 December 2011].

World Health Organization (WHO) (2011) *SAVE LIVES: Clean Your Hands.* Available on: http://www.who.int/entity/gpsc/5may/background/en/ [accessed 7 February 2011].

11

MEDICINES MANAGEMENT: INJECTION TECHNIQUE – S/C AND IM DRUG CALCULATIONS, ORAL DRUG ADMINISTRATION AND STORAGE OF MEDICINES

Matthew Aldridge

Aim

The aim of this chapter is to give an overview of the principles and storage of medications, in particular with reference to oral, subcutaneous and intramuscular routes of administration.

Objectives

- Discuss different routes of medication administration, namely:
  - oral
  - subcutaneous
  - intramuscular injections

(Continued)

(Continued)

- Describe the correct procedure for the administration of medications via the:
  - oral route
  - subcutaneous route
  - intramuscular route
- Identify key issues and steps in the safe storage and administration of medicines.

INTRODUCTION TO THE SKILL

'Medicines management' has now become a familiar term in the healthcare setting as an umbrella phrase to describe the storage, use and administration of medications. The Medicines and Healthcare Products Regulatory Authority (MHRA) 2004 offers the following definition of medicines management:

> The clinical, cost-effective and safe use of medicines to ensure patients get the maximum benefit from the medicines they need, while at the same time minimising potential harm.

The safe and effective management and administration of medications in the healthcare setting is now concurrent with the roles and responsibilities of a number of healthcare professions: nurses, doctors, pharmacists, operating department practitioners, midwives and so on. The administration of medicines is a vital component of healthcare delivery, but also one where the potential for error and harm to the patient or client exists. Therefore, it is vital that healthcare professionals have a good understanding of the legislation and practicalities surrounding the issue of medicines management, storage and administration.

BACKGROUND TO THE SKILL

The administration of medicines takes place in all healthcare settings, from primary care in the patient's home or healthcare clinic through to the complex interventions of secondary and tertiary care providers. Wherever it takes place, the same safety principles must apply to ensure maximum therapeutic benefit and minimisation of adverse effects to the patient or client.

GETTING READY TO PERFORM THE SKILL

ESSENTIAL KNOWLEDGE OF SAFE STORAGE AND SUPPLY OF MEDICINES

It is vital that the healthcare professional with a responsibility for supplying or administering medication has a good understanding of the pharmacological actions, side effects, cautions and contraindications associated with any medicines they are dealing with. If in any doubt, the healthcare professional should consult any or all of the following for clarification: the prescriber, a registered pharmacist, doctor, senior colleague or the British National Formulary (BNF).

The healthcare professional must be aware of the existing legislation governing the safe storage and supply of medicines. The principle Act regulating the supply and use of medicines in the UK is the Medicines Act 1968. This Act covers how medicines are provided to the public and is broadly categorised into:

- General sales list drugs (GSL): These may be sold to the public through general retailers. An example of this would be paracetamol from a supermarket or convenience store
- Pharmacy only (P): This classification of medicines may only be purchased under the supervision of a registered pharmacist; for example, chlorphenamine for the treatment of minor allergy from a retail pharmacy
- Prescription only: (PoM): Such medicines can only be obtained from a registered pharmacist on prescription from a registered doctor, dentist or other registered non-medical prescriber. For example, an intravenous antibiotic prescribed in the hospital setting or an oral antibiotic prescribed by a General Practitioner (GP) in the community.

It is imperative that the healthcare professional administering the drug is aware of which category of the Medicines Act 1968 that drug falls within and how they are authorised to supply or administer it in relation to their professional guidelines.

All medicines in the healthcare environment should be stored in a locked trolley/cupboard/locker or locked refrigerator, as appropriate. In compliance with the Misuse of Drugs Act (1971) and the Misuse of Drugs (Safe Custody Regulations) (1973), all drugs which appear on the controlled drugs list should be kept in a locked cupboard; the keys to which should be held at all times by an appropriate registered practitioner. All episodes of administration and receipt of new stock of controlled drugs should be administered and witnessed according to a two-person system.

The use of patient group directives (PGDs) has gained popularity in a number of healthcare settings in recent years, including hospitals, private clinics and custodial settings. A PGD allows a registered practitioner, following additional training, to administer certain approved drugs to previously unnamed patients or clients without a direct prescription. This can be useful where a patient or client requires a drug but access to an authorised prescriber may be delayed. An example of this is a triage nurse in an Emergency Department administering paracetamol to a patient presenting with a minor injury while they wait to be seen by a doctor. The PGD must have been drawn up in agreement with a doctor and registered pharmacist, and will function only in agreement with the organisation in which it is to be used. The person administering the drug must ensure that the patient/client fulfils the category for the use of the PGD, and has no allergies or contraindications to the drug to be administered. For registered nurses, it is important to note that only the person designated to administer a drug under a PGD is allowed to do so and this task may not be delegated, for example, to a student nurse under the supervision of such a registered nurse (NMC, 2008).

DRUG CALCULATIONS

The administration of medications requiring the calculation of dosages has been identified as a particular source of error (Fry and Dacey, 2007; National Patient Safety Agency, 2009; McMullan, 2010). For this reason, it is imperative that healthcare professionals who have a responsibility for the prescription and administration of medicines are familiar with the application of the appropriate formulae for dosage calculations. Some of the more commonly used formulae appear in Box 11.1.

BOX 11.1   COMMON DRUG CALCULATION FORMULAE

To Calculate a Drug Volume from Stock Strength

What you want / what you have got × volume

Example:

> Pethidine IM 50mg is prescribed; stock dose is 75mg in 3ml
> 50 / 75 × 3 = 2ml of Pethidine to be drawn up

Gravity-feed intravenous infusions

Volume / time (in hours) × drops per ml the giving set delivers/minutes (60) = drops per minute (dpm)

Example:

> 1000mls of normal saline to be given over four hours
> 1000 / 4 = 250; 20/60 = 0.33; 250 × 0.33 = 83 drops per minute

Note: crystalloid giving sets usually deliver 20 drops/ml and colloid/blood giving sets 15 drops/ml (always check the packaging before use to confirm the delivery rate).

If the infusion is to be given in less than an hour the following formula can be used:

Volume of infusion (ml) × drops per ml of administration set/number of minutes infusion is set to run

Electronic pump intravenous infusions

Volume of infusion (ml) / time (hours) = ml per hour

Example:

> 1000mls of normal saline to be given over two hours
> 1000 / 2 = 500 ml per hour

Weight related doses

Prescribed dose × body weight = dose

Example:

   1mg of clexane per Kg of body weight (70kg)
   $1 \times 70 = 70$mg of clexane to be administered

NB All answers should be rounded to the nearest whole number, for example, '53.6 drops per minute' would be '54 drops per minute' when rounded to the nearest whole number.

FIVE RIGHTS OF DRUG ADMINISTRATION

The healthcare professional with a responsibility for the administration of medicines should at all times follow the systematic steps associated with safe drug administration, as detailed by the Department of Health (DH) (2004) and Nursing and Midwifery Council (NMC), (2008), commonly referred to as the 'Five Rights' or 'Five Rs' of drug administration. These are:

- Right patient: by ensuring that the details on the patient's identification bracelet, and preferably by verbal confirmation with the patient, match those on the prescription
- Right drug: check the external packaging and internal packaging (e.g. blister pack) to verify drug name against the details of the prescription – check with BNF or other sources if unsure
- Right dose: check packaging for drug dose, check with other sources as above to verify if necessary, and ensure correct calculation of dose using appropriate formulae if drug is not presented in the dose required
- Right route: check packaging, prescription and details of the patient's condition for the indicated route
- Right time: check the prescription, and the BNF if necessary, for indicated frequencies of administration.

PROCEDURES FOR DRUG ADMINISTRATION

We shall now discuss in turn the administration of medicine via the oral, intramuscular and subcutaneous routes.

ORAL DRUG ADMINISTRATION: PERFORMING THE SKILL

POINTS TO NOTE

Abbreviations can be potentially confusing and a source of error; however, it is important that those professionals with a responsibility for the administration of

Table 11.1

Action	Rationale
Ensure that local policies and guidelines are followed on the administration of medicines	To ensure that medication is being administered in the safest way possible
Prepare the necessary equipment for administration, i.e. mobile drugs trolley and prescription sheet or electronic prescribing records	To ensure that the process is carried out correctly and smoothly
Perform appropriate hand hygiene as per local protocol	To prevent transmission of infection when administering oral medication
The timing of ward drug administration rounds is important and protected time should be allowed for the practitioner to carry out this task (Fry and Dacey, 2007)	To minimise distractions and interruptions to the practitioner which could lead to maladministration or error
Ensure that baseline patient assessment and observations have been carried out prior to administration of medicines	In order to prevent hypersensitivity and adverse reactions, such as the contraindication to administer digoxin to the bradycardic patient
Explain to patient and obtain consent	Medication administration should be an open process, fully involving the patient to promote benefit and gain compliance
Is the patient/client able to swallow sufficiently well to take the medicine offered? If there is any question as to a patient's swallowing status, i.e. following a neurological insult such as CVA, then the input of a speech and language therapist should be sought and the prescriber informed as soon as possible	To prevent potential choking or aspiration incidents if the patient has dysphagia. If swallowing is impaired, an alternative route should be sought
Check the prescription chart or electronic prescribing record for any due medications	To ensure administration is in accordance with the prescription
Perform the 'Five rights' of medication administration as detailed above; Right patient, Right drug, Right route, Right dose, Right time	To prevent maladministration of the medication

(Continued)

Table 11.1   (Continued)

Action	Rationale
Tip the required amount of capsules, tablets or liquids into an appropriate container, e.g. a medicine 'tot'. Tablets should first be tipped into the lid of the container and blister packs should be pressed through from the back of the blister strip	Medicines should not be handled directly to promote infection control principles and reduce exposure of certain substances to the person administering the medication
Note: syringes intended for intravenous use should not be used for measuring oral medication (NPSA, 2007). Special syringes intended only for oral/enteral use are available, labelled as such and colour-coded purple	To prevent the inadvertent intravenous administration of an oral medication to a patient/client
Oral capsules and tablets should not be crushed or broken, unless specifically directed to do by the drug manufacturer or a registered pharmacist. If the patient/client is unable to take a medication in capsule/tablet form, then an alternative should be sought such as oral liquid suspension	Breaking or crushing a capsule or tablet may alter its chemical and pharmacological properties, thus potentially rendering it ineffective or harmful. It is safer to get the drug re-prescribed and dispensed as an oral liquid suspension which the patient may find easier or more palatable to swallow
The healthcare professional with responsibility for medication administration should remain with the patient/client until they are satisfied that the medication has been swallowed	If the healthcare professional does not observe the patient/client swallowing the drug, it may not be administered due to the patient/client forgetting, or potentially the drug may be taken accidentally or otherwise by another patient/client
The administration of medication should be appropriately recorded on the prescription chart or electronic prescribing record immediately after administration. If for any reason the medication was not administered, this should be recorded and reported as per local protocol	This provides a permanent record that the drug has been administered and is necessary for continuity of care
The practitioner should periodically observe the patient/client for any adverse effects of the medication once administered	So that any adverse drug reaction (ADR) can be detected, reported and acted upon

medications are familiar with the accepted abbreviations used in the prescribing of medicines. A list of common abbreviations (British National Formulary (BNF), 2010) appears in Table 11. 2.

Table 11.2

Abbreviation	Explanation
a. c.	ante cibum (before food)
b. d.	bis die (twice daily)
o. d.	omni die (every day)
o. m.	omni mane (every morning)
o. n.	omni nocte (every night)
p. c.	post cibum (after food)
p. r. n.	pro re nata (when required)
q. d. s.	quater die sumendum (to be taken four times daily)
q. q. h.	quarta quaque hora (every four hours)
stat	immediately
t. d. s.	ter die sumendum (to be taken three times daily)
t. i. d.	ter in die (three times daily)

The issue of covert drug administration (giving of medications without the patient's knowledge or consent) should be discussed. It should also be noted that this procedure is to be avoided, as it is considered to be undesirable, unless absolutely unavoidable and in the patient's best interest (Nursing and Midwifery Concil (NMC), 2008).

Never administer a medicine that you have not prepared yourself. This can introduce a significant risk of error if the practitioner administering the drug has not checked the packaging and dose preparation for themselves.

INTRAMUSCULAR INJECTION

An intramuscular injection involves the delivery of a medicine (injectate) directly into a muscle, whereby it can be absorbed rapidly (Shawyer and Endacott, 2009, in Endacott et al., 2009). The advantages of intramuscular injections (IM) are that they are quickly absorbed (within 20 minutes) and can be used to inject substances which may otherwise irritate the subcutaneous tissue (Greenway, 2004).

SITE FOR INJECTION

There are five widely accepted sites for the delivery of intramuscular injection (Rodger and King, 2000) as highlighted in Table 11.3.

NEEDLE SIZE AND SELECTION

The needle selected should be able to penetrate through the subcutaneous layer into the muscle tissue; hence at least a blue needle (23G) will be required (Shawyer and Endacott, 2009). However, for patients/clients with larger adipose tissues layers, a green needle (21G) may be required. The drug to be administered should be drawn up with no larger than a green needle (21G) as any needle larger than this increases the risk of unwanted particulates being drawn up from the ampoule into the syringe, particularly if glass ampoules are involved. The needle should always be changed after the drawing-up of a drug and replaced with a new needle to administer the drug. This is done to minimise the risk of injecting particulates which may have been

Table 11.3

Muscle site	Amount that can be injected (mls)
Dorsogluteal: upper outer quadrant of buttock. A risk of penetrating the sciatic nerve or gluteal arteries exists, therefore this technique is less commonly recommended for routine injections (WHO, 2004)	Up to maximum of 4 ml
Rectus femoris: anterior (front) middle of thigh, quadriceps muscle	Up to a maximum of 5 ml
Vastus lateralis: lateral (outer) aspect of thigh in quadriceps area	Up to a maximum of 5 ml
Ventrogluteal: upper thigh over greater trochanter area	Up to a maximum of 2.5ml
Deltoid: upper outer aspect of arm (more commonly used for immunisations due to ease of access and low volumes of injectate to be administered)	Up to a maximum of 1ml

drawn-up into the needle, and also because the tip of the needle may have become blunted while drawing up which would, potentially, increase discomfort for the patient/client during the procedure.

Z-TRACK TECHNIQUE

The Z-track technique of intramuscular injection involves the practitioner manually displacing the skin and subcutaneous tissue on a patient's limb by pulling the skin and tissue laterally prior to administering the injection (Rodger and King, 2000). The skin and subcutaneous tissue is then immediately released as soon as the injection has been administered. This has the benefit of sealing the medication into the muscle tissue and preventing leakage into the subcutaneous area. This can be particularly useful when administering medications which may be an irritant to skin and subcutaneous tissue.

INTRAMUSCULAR INJECTION: PERFORMING THE SKILL

POINTS TO NOTE

Consider the use of alternative devices such as 'auto-injector' devices, for example, the EpiPen™ which is used by patients/clients in an emergency situation to self-administer adrenaline for the treatment of anaphylaxis. Also to be discussed or demonstrated, if deemed appropriate, are 'auto-disable' devices whereby the needle retracts into the syringe housing following injection in an attempt to reduce the risk of needle-stick injury to the operator. Rehearsal of injection technique skill can be carried out on proprietary part-task training devices or 'injection pads' which are designed to replicate the feel of human tissue. Alternatively it is possible to practise the injection technique with a piece of fruit such as an orange, which allows a reasonable level of fidelity in terms of tactile feedback of the procedure for the student.

SUBCUTANEOUS INJECTION

Subcutaneous injection involves the administration of a medication beneath the epidermis into the underlying fat and connective tissue. This mode of injection is particularly useful when small volumes of medication, typically less than 2ml (Nicol et al., 2008), requiring a slow absorption rate, are to be administered. Common drugs administered via the subcutaneous route include insulin and low-molecular weight heparins for the prophylaxis and treatment of thrombus formation. Any drug administered via this route should be highly soluble in order to prevent irritation to tissue (Dougherty and Lister, 2008).

Table 11.4

Action	Rationale
Ensure that local policies and guidelines are followed on the administration of medicines	To ensure that medication is being administered in the safest way possible
Perform appropriate hand hygiene as per local protocol	To minimise risk of cross-infection
Prepare the necessary equipment for administration: syringe (appropriate dose, i.e. 2ml or 5ml syringe)	To ensure that the process is carried out correctly and smoothly
Two needles: one for drawing up of medication and one for administration	
Plastic tray (receiver) first cleansed with an alcohol cleansing solution	To carry injection to patient and prevent cross-contamination
Alcohol swab	If the site on patient's skin requires cleansing
Sharps disposal bin	For safe sharps disposal
Gauze or cotton wool	In case of bleeding post-injection
Introduce yourself to the patient, explain the procedure and gain consent	To ensure the patient understands the procedure and agrees to it
Position the patient accordingly and adjust their clothing, i.e. if the injection is to be given in the thigh the patient should be lying down with limb exposed, while maintaining patient dignity at all times	To promote patient comfort and compliance and maintain patient's privacy and dignity when clothing is adjusted/removed
Assess the skin around the intended injection site to ensure that there are no broken areas, lesions or signs of infection. Avoid repeated injection around the same site	To avoid the risk of introducing a localised infection systemically and avoid complications. Injection sites should be rotated to prevent hardening of the tissues which may affect absorption of the drug
Perform the 'Five rights' of medication administration: Right patient, Right drug, Right route, Right dose, Right time	To prevent maladministration of the medicine
Identify injection site and landmarks on patient's limb, as appropriate	To ensure correct intramuscular injection technique is followed

(Continued)

Table 11.4   (Continued)

Action	Rationale
Cleaning the skin with an alcohol-based wipe is only required if the area is visibly dirty or the patient is immunocompromised	Research demonstrates that routine skin cleansing has no benefit before IM injection (Department of Health, 2006)
Hold the syringe between thumb and index finger (keeping thumb off the plunger), inserting the needle with a smooth, swift action at a 90 degree angle into the correct site (see Figure 11.1)	Ensure thumb is kept away from plunger whilst inserting the needle to avoid early administration into the subcutaneous tissue
Pull back on plunger slightly to check for the presence of blood in syringe. If no blood visualised, inject medication at the rate of approximately 1ml of fluid over 10 seconds (Dougherty and Lister, 2008). If blood appears in syringe, withdraw, discard needle and syringe, start procedure afresh	Check for the presence of blood to avoid inadvertent administration of medication into a blood vessel rather than muscle
Once drug is injected, pause for 10 seconds before withdrawing needle	To allow time for drug to diffuse and prevent leakage
Withdraw needle quickly and smoothly, dispose of needle in sharps container immediately. Never re-sheath a used needle	To minimise patient discomfort To prevent needle-stick injury and ensure safe disposal Re-sheathing a used needle poses a significant risk of needle-stick injury
Observe injection site for bleeding and apply pressure accordingly if bleeding observed. Do not rub the site of injection	To prevent haemorrhage or haematoma formation at site of injection Rubbing may encourage bleeding/ haematoma and increase patient discomfort
Sign for administration of drug on patient's prescription chart or electronic prescription and update patient's notes accordingly	To maintain an accurate record and ensure continuity of care
Dispose of any other waste as appropriate and wash hands	To minimise risk of cross-infection
The practitioner should periodically observe the patient/client for any adverse effects of the medication once administered	So that any adverse drug reaction (ADR) can be detected, reported and acted upon

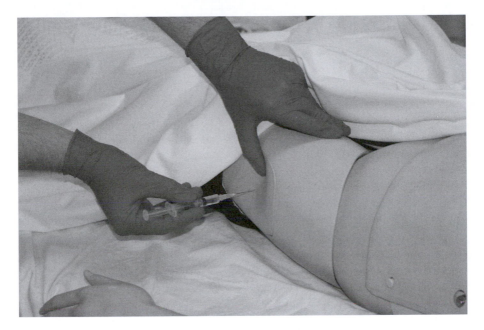

Figure 11.1

NEEDLE SIZE AND SELECTION

Some drugs to be administered via the subcutaneous route will be pre-packaged in their own syringe with needle attached, typically a fine gauge needle. If this is to be used then the practitioner should pinch the patient's/client's skin into a fold and insert the needle into the patient at a 90 degree angle to ensure adequate penetration of the subcutaneous layer. If an Orange 25G needle is to be used, where the drug is not presented in a pre-filled syringe and requires being drawn-up from an ampoule, then the practitioner should pinch the patient's/client's skin and insert the needle at 45 degrees to prevent further penetration beyond the subcutaneous tissue.

SITES FOR INJECTION

The following three sites are commonly used for the administration of subcutaneous injection (Hunter, 2008):

- Lateral aspect of the thigh area
- Umbilical region of the abdomen
- Outer aspect of the upper arm.

SUBCUTANEOUS INJECTION: PERFORMING THE SKILL

Table 11.5

Action	Rationale
Ensure that local policies and guidelines are followed on the administration of medicines	To ensure that medication is being administered in the safest way possible
Perform appropriate hand hygiene as per local protocol	To minimise risk of cross-infection
Position the patient according to the injection site chosen and adjust their clothing, i.e. if the injection is to be given in the thigh, the patient should be lying down with limb exposed, while maintaining patient dignity at all times	To promote patient comfort and compliance and maintain patient's privacy and dignity when clothing is adjusted/removed
Prepare the necessary equipment for administration:	
Syringe appropriate to drug volume, i.e. 2ml Or drug in pre-packaged syringe if appropriate	To ensure the use of appropriate resource
Orange (25G) needle to draw up and administer drug if not in pre-packaged syringe and Orange (25G) needle to administer the drug	Needle should be changed between drawing-up and administering drug to minimise patient discomfort
Plastic tray (receiver) first cleansed with alcohol-based solution	To carry equipment to patient's/client's bedside and minimise the risk of cross-infection
Sharps container	For safe disposal of sharps
Patient's prescription sheet/ electronic prescription record	To cross-check patient and drug details
Assess the skin around the intended injection site to ensure that there are no broken areas, lesions or signs of infection. Avoid repeated injection around the same site	To avoid the risk of introducing a localised infection systemically and avoid complications. Injection sites should be rotated to prevent hardening of the tissues which may affect absorption of the drug

(Continued)

Table 11.5   (Continued)

Action	Rationale
Perform the 'Five rights' of medication administration as detailed above: Right patient, Right drug, Right route, Right dose, Right time	To prevent maladministration of the medicine
Gently pinch the skin into a fold in the area to be injected	To gather the subcutaneous tissue together
Insert the needle with a smooth, swift motion into the area to be injected; either at 90 degrees if a short needle on a pre-packaged syringe, or 45 degrees if using an Orange (25G) needle (see Figure 11.2)	Correct angle for needle size is important to ensure successful infiltration of the subcutaneous tissue only
There is no need to pull back on the plunger to check for blood before commencing injection	The capillary network around the subcutaneous tissue is too fine to risk accidental intravenous administration
Depress the plunger of the syringe and inject the medication slowly	To aid distribution of the drug into the subcutaneous layer and minimise the risk of bruising
Withdraw the needle in a smooth motion and check the injection site for bleeding (apply gauze or cotton wool if necessary)	
Do not rub the injection site	In order to minimise the risk of bruising and discomfort to the patient

POINTS TO NOTE

A demonstration of subcutaneous injection administration equipment should also include the use of 'insulin pen' delivery systems, which come as a self-contained unit requiring the user to change the variable dose via a dial, usually at the end of the device. This requires careful manipulation to ensure that the correct dose is delivered every time, and is a necessary focus for health promotion/education in those patients/clients who will be self-administering insulin away from the clinical setting.

There are also important differences to note with pre-filled medications for subcutaneous injections, namely: the shorter needle length (requiring a 90 degree

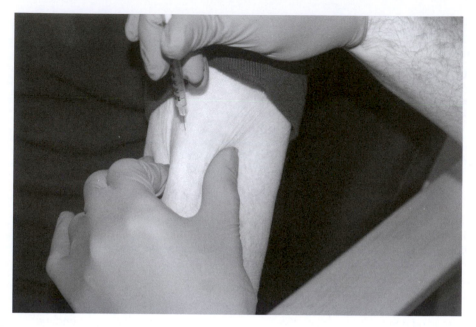

Figure 11.2

angle of attack) and the fact that the air in a pre-filled syringe next to the plunger should not be expelled prior to injection, as this ensures that the correct dose of the medication is administered.

CONCLUSION – A SUMMARY OF IMPORTANT POINTS ABOUT THE SKILL

The skill of drug administration is more than the physical act of passing medicine to a patient or client. It requires the practitioner to be knowledgeable about the indications, side effects and pharmacological actions of a drug. It is also vital that any practitioner with responsibility for the administration of medications has an understanding of the legislation surrounding medication supply and storage.

In order for any practitioner to be confident and competent in the administration of medication, opportunity for rehearsal of the skill in a supervised environment is essential. Simulation lends itself to the acquisition of medication administration skills as it allows the practitioner to familiarise themselves with and manipulate the equipment to be used. Simulation also allows the learner to practise the administration of medications with either manikins or role players (Standardised Patients), thus reducing harm to actual patients in this critical phase of care delivery.

Covert Administration of Medication

Aim

- For the learner to gain a practical understanding of the issues faced when dealing with the issue of covert administration of medication to a patient/client.

Objectives

At the end of this simulation the student will be able to:

- Analyse and discuss the relevant legislation and guidance when faced with the potential of covert drug administration
- Demonstrate an understanding of the ethical and practical issues of covert drug administration/crushing of oral medication
- Demonstrate strategies for safe oral medication administration.

Aids to Support Compliance

NMC Standards for Medicine Management 2008 Standard 16

Registrants must assess the patient's suitability and understanding of how to use an appropriate compliance aid safely.

Crushing Medication

The mechanics of crushing medicines may alter their therapeutic properties rendering them ineffective and are not covered by their product licence (Barber and Robertson, 2009). Medicinal products should not routinely be crushed unless a pharmacist advises that the medication is not compromised by crushing, and crushing has been determined to be within the patient's best interest.

Disguising Medication

As a general principle, by disguising medication in food or drink, the patient or client is being led to believe they are not receiving medication when, in fact, they are. The NMC would not consider this to be good practice. The registrant would need to be sure what they are doing is *in the best interests of the patient* and be aware that they are accountable for this decision. See the NMC A–Z of advice for further information (www.nmc-uk.org).

This scenario addresses the issue of crushing up medication, the disguising of medication and the challenging of senior staff members' practice.

This scenario can be re-run several times in quick succession with different students.

Equipment/Resources Required

- Role player (standardised patient) briefed to act as patient
- Role player to act as Registered nurse undertaking drug round

- Drugs trolley
- Drug prescription chart
- Medication tot
- Two spoons
- Patient's lunch plate
- Placebo drugs or sweets intended to represent oral tablets.

Setting

Hospital ward drug round, 12.00hrs
   Patient bedside
   NB: scenario could be easily modified to a community setting or nursing/residential home setting.

Situation

A student nurse is accompanying an experienced staff nurse on a drug round. On approaching the next patient, the staff nurse begins to crush tablets and states they will mix them into the patient's dinner as he is awkward. The nurse will ask the student to mix them into the dinner. The student will have to react to the situation, identifying potentially unsafe practice.

Roles

Table 11.6

Staff Nurse	Role to be taken by facilitator. When starting the next patient's administration you begin to crush tablets and state that they will mix them into the patient's dinner as he is 'awkward'. Then you as the nurse will ask the student to mix them into the dinner. Be very persuasive and, if challenged, state that you have been doing this for years and it doesn't do anyone any harm. Eventually back down if the student gives you a good reason for not crushing the tablets
Student Nurse	Role to be taken by a student nurse. You are on a drug round with a more experienced staff nurse

Areas for Discussion

- Patient consent
- Who is the nurse crushing the tablets for, the patient or for their own convenience?
- See Standard 16 above
- How did the student deal with this?
- How should we challenge poor practice?

REFERENCES

Barber, P. and Robertson, D. (2009) *Essentials of Pharmacology for Nurses*. Berkshire: Open University Press, McGraw-Hill Education. p. 162.

British National Formulary (Joint Formulary Committee) (2010) *60th Edition*. London: British Medical Association and Royal Pharmaceutical Society.

Department of Health (DH) (2004) *Building a Safer NHS for Patients: Improving Medication Safety*. London: HMSO.

Department of Health (DH) (2006) *Immunisation against Infectious Disease – The Green Book*. London: The Stationery Office.

Dougherty, L. and Lister, S. (2008) *The Royal Marsden Hospital Manual of Clinical Nursing Procedures*, 7th edn. London: Wiley-Blackwell.

Endacott, R., Jevon, P. and Cooper, S. (2009) *Clinical Nursing Skills: Core and Advanced*. Oxford: Oxford University Press.

Fry, M.M. and Dacey, C. (2007) 'Factors contributing to incidents in medicine administration: part 2', *British Journal of Nursing*, 16 (11): 676–81.

Greenway, K. (2004) 'Using the ventrogluteal site for intramuscular injections', *Nursing Standard*, 18 (25): 39–42.

Hunter, J. (2008) 'Subcutaneous injection technique', *Nursing Standard*, 22 (21): 42.

McMullan, M. (2010) 'Exploring the numeracy skills of nurses and students when performing drug calculations', *Nursing Times*, 106 (34): 10–12.

Medicines Act (1968) London: HMSO.

Medicine and Healthcare Products Regulatory Authority (MHRA) (2004) cited in Nursing and Midwifery Council (2008) *Standards for Medicines Management*. London: NMC.

Misuse of Drugs Act (1971) London: HMSO.

Misuse of Drugs (Safe Custody Regulations) Act (1973) London: HMSO.

National Patient Safety Agency (NPSA) (2007) *Patient Safety Alert 19: Promoting Safer Measurement and Administration of Liquid Medicines via Oral and Other Enteral Routes*. London: NPSA.

National Patient Safety Agency (NPSA) (2009) *Review of Patient Safety for Children and Young People*. London: NPSA.

National Prescribing Centre (2001) *Modernising Medicines Management: A Guide to Achieving Benefits for Patients, Professionals and the NHS*. Liverpool: National Prescribing Centre and National Primary Care Research and Development Centre.

Nicol, M., Bavin, C., Cronin, P. and Rawlings-Anderson, K. (2008) *Essential Nursing Skills*, 3rd edn. London: Mosby Elsevier.

Nursing and Midwifery Council (NMC) (2008) *Standards for Medicines Management*. London: NMC.

Rodger, M. and King, L. (2000) 'Drawing up and administering intramuscular injections: a review of the literature', *Journal of Advanced Nursing*, 13: 574–82.

Shawyer, V. and Endacott, R. (2009) 'Administering an intramuscular injection', in R. Endacott, P. Jevon and S. Cooper (eds), *Clinical Nursing Skills: Core and Advanced*. Oxford: Oxford University Press.

World Health Organization (WHO) (2004) *Immunization in Practice: Module 6 Holding an Immunization Session*. Geneva: WHO.

12

RESPIRATORY CARE: O^2 THERAPY, PULSE OXIMETRY AND INHALED MEDICATION

Catherine Easthope, Philip Jevon and Steven Webb

Aim

The aim of this chapter is to understand how to provide simulation training in the teaching of respiratory skills.

Chapter Objectives

At the end of this chapter the reader will be able to provide simulation in:

- Peak expiratory flow measurement
- Use of a metered dose inhaler
- Use of a spacer device
- Use of a nebuliser
- Use of a non-rebreathe mask
- Pulse oximetry.

PEAK EXPIRATORY FLOW MEASUREMENT

INTRODUCTION

Peak expiratory flow (PEF), also called the peak expiratory flow rate (PEFR), can be defined as a person's maximum speed of expiration. It measures the airflow through the bronchi and thus the degree of obstruction in the airways.

The measurement of peak expiratory flow was pioneered by Dr Martin Wright, who produced the first meter to measure the lung function. It was originally introduced in the late 1950s, since when it has developed into the simplest, quickest and cheapest test of lung function. It is more useful in the monitoring of patients with established asthma than in making the initial diagnosis (British Thoracic Society and SIGN, 2008).

Healthcare professionals need to be aware that peak flow measurement is dependant upon patient effort and technique, which is key to obtaining an acceptable reading. It should be used as a guide to management in patients with established asthma and a good history of the patient's symptoms needs to be taken to complement the peak flow reading.

BACKGROUND

Since 2004 peak flow meters in the UK have had to comply with a new European standard (EN 13826) for measuring the peak expiratory flow. Some patients and healthcare professionals may still be using the old scale meters and it is, therefore, important to ensure that the meter is checked to make sure it adheres to the EU standard. Normal expected values of peak flow depend on the patient's sex, age and height. It is measured in litres per minute (L/Min).

There are two types of peak flow meters, low and standard range:

- Standard range peak flow meters are suitable for both adults and children over six years of age (under-six-year-olds can get confused about inhalation and expiration)
- Low range peak flow meters are designed for adults and children with severely impaired function of the lungs.

The peak flow is a good measurement of a patient's lung function for healthcare professionals. It can be the main clinical indicator to highlight uncontrolled asthma as the readings could change a lot from day to day or between morning and evening. When asthma is well controlled, there should be little difference in the day-to-day peak flow measurement.

The patient would first need to find out what their normal readings should be. The highest peak flow, when the asthma is well controlled, will usually be taken as the normal reading.

Within the ward environment, the peak flow is a good guide to the patient's progress and it is essential that all patients with asthma have peak flow charts and that their peak flow is recorded daily. The number of times it is recorded per day will depend on local policy. The peak flow test should be carried out three times and the highest result of the three plotted on the peak flow chart. The same advice would be given to a patient who is at home and carrying out their own peak flow measurements. The peak flow is usually done twice daily, with the best times for testing being between 6 and 8 a.m. prior to inhaler dose and then between 4 and 5 p.m.

Patients at home should also list daily the symptoms they are experiencing as this will give their general practitioner or practice nurse a better idea of control. It is important that patients at home and who carry out peak flows are given a detailed asthma self-management plan by an appropriately trained healthcare professional. This will allow the patient to continue to monitor their peak flows and alter their medications to achieve control if their peak flow falls below their personal best. The plan is individual to that patient and should be clear. Always ensure you provide a written copy for them to keep.

GETTING READY TO PERFORM THE SKILL

1   The healthcare professional will need to ensure that they have a peak flow meter that complies with the EU standards. The peak flow meters are single patient use and should be left with that patient once peak flows are initiated.
2   The healthcare professional needs to ensure they have the appropriate peak flow charts so that the result can be recorded immediately.
3   The procedure needs to be explained to the patient and an explanation given of why the peak flow is an important part of their management.
4   Verbal consent should be obtained prior to commencement.
5   Ideally the peak flow should be performed standing but can be done with the patient sitting in an upright position, in a comfortable chair with arms.

PROCEDURE

- Check that the pointer is at zero
- Preferably stand or sit in a comfortable, upright position
- Hold the peak flow meter level (horizontally) and keep the fingers away from the pointer
- Take a deep breath and close the lips firmly around the mouthpiece
- Blow as hard as you can – as if you were blowing out candles on a birthday cake – remember it's the speed of the blow that is measured
- Look at the pointer and check the reading
- Reset the pointer back to zero
- This should be repeated twice more and the highest reading recorded.

CONCLUSION

Peak flow recording is a guide to the patient's management and should be done in conjunction with a clear, concise history of symptoms. It should be accompanied by an asthma self-management plan which has been personalised for that patient and written by a qualified healthcare professional.

Remember that peak flows are technique dependant and can be variable, so the person assessing the skill should encourage good technique and record poor technique. It could be appropriate to demonstrate the technique to a patient rather than explain it to them in words.

METERED DOSE INHALER

INTRODUCTION

The metered dose inhaler (MDI) is a device used to administer a drug straight into the lungs as the patient inhales. It is the cheapest and most commonly used inhaler. It requires good coordination and a good technique, which is essential for optimal drug deposition within the lungs. The MDI is a pressurised metal canister which holds the drug and a liquid propellant. As it states, it administers a metered dose of the drug to the patient in aerosol form.

The inhaler is usually used in conditions such as asthma and chronic obstructive pulmonary disease (COPD). Technique is essential to maintain health and control the patient's symptoms. It is the healthcare professional's responsibility to observe inhaler technique and ensure that it is used in the correct way. In a recent study, patients with uncontrolled asthma were assessed on their ability to use a metered dose inhaler. Of the 2,123 patients reviewed, 1,092 failed to use the inhaler correctly. After instruction they found a significant increase in good technique (Hardwell et al., 2009).

BACKGROUND

The first metered dose inhaler was developed in 1955 by Riker Laboratories although there is documented evidence of the inhalation of medicines via devices as early as the 17th century.

Cooordination and dexterity are an intrinsic factor in the patient's ability to be able to use the inhaler device correctly and for the long-term management of respiratory disease. At every opportunity the healthcare professional should assess the patient. There are a number of devices available and aids which can complement those devices. For the purpose of this skill we shall concentrate on the metered dose inhaler, the most popular of all inhalers but possibly one of the most difficult to use.

GETTING READY TO PERFORM THE SKILL

- The healthcare professional will need to introduce themselves and explain to the patient what they intend to do and the benefits of a good technique
- The healthcare professional needs to ensure that they have a placebo device available so that they can demonstrate the correct technique to the patient prior to assessment of the patient's own technique
- Verbal consent should be obtained prior to commencement
- The patient should be in a comfortable position
- It may be useful to have some written information about the technique which the patient could take away with them at the end, to reinforce the technique.

STEP–BY-STEP APPROACH – PROCEDURE

- Remove the cap
- Shake the inhaler
- Breathe out gently, so the lungs are emptied and maximum inhalation can be achieved
- Put the mouthpiece in the mouth and at the start of an inspiration, which should be slow and deep, press the canister and continue to inhale
- Hold the breath for 10 seconds, or as long as possible, and then breathe out slowly
- Wait a few seconds before repeating the steps above
- Replace the cap.

CONCLUSION

Inhalers are an essential part of treatment for a respiratory patient and the patient's technique should be assessed at every consultation to ensure management of the disease is maintained. Although the metered dose inhaler is the most common of all, it is essential that the healthcare professional is able to demonstrate use of all inhalers to ensure the patient has a variety of devices to choose from. This is important as good technique will, in turn, facilitate treatments compliance.

USE OF A SPACER DEVICE

INTRODUCTION

A spacer device is a large plastic or metal container, with a mouthpiece at one end and a hole for the aerosol inhaler at the other (Asthma UK, 2007). It is basically a chamber that acts as a reservoir for the aerosol cloud (see Figure 12.1 for an image of a spacer being used), removing the need for coordinating actuation of a metered dose inhaler (MDI) and inhalation (Pearce, 2000).

A spacer device will only work with an aerosol inhaler (Asthma UK, 2007). When used correctly, an MDI with a spacer device attached is at least as effective as any other device for delivering inhaled drugs (Currie and Douglas, 2007). The spacer is a useful substitute for a nebuliser in the treatment of acute asthma (Rees and Kanabar, 2006).

TYPES OF SPACER DEVICES

There are several spacer devices currently available, though the larger ones with a one-way valve (for example, Nebulaher and Volumatic) are the most effective (British Medical Association and Royal Pharmaceutical Society of Great Britain, 2010).

ADVANTAGES OF USING A SPACER DEVICE

Advantages of using a spacer device include:

- Making aerosol inhalers easier to use: removes the need for coordination between actuation of an MDI and inhalation
- Reducing the velocity of the aerosol and subsequent impaction on the patient's oropharynx
- Allowing more time for the propellant to evaporate, thus enabling a larger proportion of the drug particles to be inhaled and deposited in the lungs
- Reducing the risk of side effects from the higher doses of preventer medicines by reducing the amount of medicine that is swallowed and absorbed into the body. (*Sources*: British Medical Association and Royal Pharmaceutical Society of Great Britain, 2010; Asthma UK, 2007).

INDICATIONS

Indications for using a spacer device include:

- Patients with poor inhaler technique
- Children and infants
- Patients requiring high doses of medications
- Nocturnal asthma
- Patients who are prone to candidiasis (oral thrush) with inhaled corticosteroids.

PRINCIPLES OF USING A SPACER

- The spacer should be compatible with the MDI that is being used
- The drug should be administered by repeated single actuations of the metered dose inhaler into the spacer, each followed by an inhalation
- There should be minimal delay between MDI actuation and inhalation
- Tidal breathing is just as effective as single breaths
- Spacers should be cleaned monthly rather than weekly as per manufacturer's recommendations or performance will be adversely affected (British Thoracic Society and Scottish Intercollegiate Network, 2008).

PROCEDURE FOR USING A SPACER DEVICE

- Ensure the spacer device is compatible to the MDI being used
- If necessary, assemble the spacer device (some devices come in two halves)
- Shake the MDI
- Remove the cap from the mouthpiece on the MDI and fit the MDI to the spacer device
- Close lips and teeth around mouthpiece
- Actuate the MDI
- Inhale deeply and slowly; ask the patient to hold their breath for 10 seconds (or as long as it is comfortable) – inhalation should be as soon as possible following actuation, definitely within 30 seconds (Rees and Kanabar, 2006)

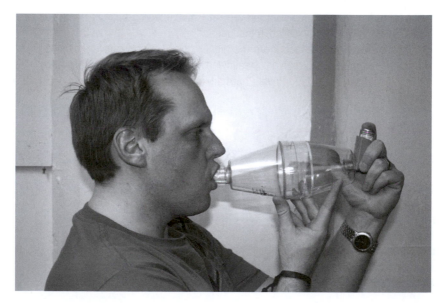

Figure 12.1

- Remove the device from the mouth and close lips
- Breathe out slowly (Asthma UK, 2007). It is recommended to take at least two deeply held breaths for each puff of the inhaler (Asthma UK, 2007). Some patients may find it difficult to take deep breaths – normal tidal breathing is considered just as effective (Asthma UK, 2007)
- If a second dose is required, wait 30–60 seconds before repeating the above procedure (Pearce, 2000)
- In infants and children under two years of age, attach a mask to the spacer device to facilitate its effective use; also hold the spacer at an angle of 45 degrees to keep the valve open – the medication can then be inhaled during normal tidal breathing (Rees and Kanabar, 2006).

USE OF A NEBULISER

INTRODUCTION

A nebuliser is a device for creating a mist of drug particles that can be inhaled via a face mask (Currie and Douglas, 2007); the word is taken from the Latin word 'nebula' meaning mist. In the healthcare setting a nebuliser is a small device that can convert a drug from a solution into aerosol form by means of a compressor/compressed gas source (Jevon, 2007a).

Nebulisation is the method of creating a mist of drug particles that can be inhaled via a facemask or a mouthpiece (Currie and Douglas, 2007). The most common nebulised drugs are bronchodilators, although many other drugs can be nebulised, for example, steroids and antibiotics.

HOW A NEBULISER WORKS

The conventional nebuliser works by a flow of gas (oxygen or air) passing through a very small hole (venturi); rapid expansion of air causes a negative pressure which sucks the nebulised fluid up the feeding tube system where it is atomised and inhaled (O'Callaghan and Barry, 1997). This passage of gas can be generated by a compressor (air) or an oxygen flow source.

The proportion of the nebulised solution that actually reaches the lungs is *approximately 12%* (Rees and Kanabar, 2006), which is the reason why *nebulised doses of drugs are higher* than doses administered via an aerosol inhaler.

MEDICATIONS THAT CAN BE ADMINISTERED VIA A NEBULISER

Medications that are commonly administered through a nebuliser include bronchodilators (e.g. salbutamol), anticholinergics (e.g. ipratropium bromide), corticosteroids (e.g. beclometasone) and normal saline.

INDICATIONS

The main indications for a nebuliser are to deliver:

- A bronchodilator or anticholinergic drug to a patient with an acute exacerbation of asthma or chronic obstructive airway disease (COPD)
- A bronchodilator or anticholinergic drug regularly to a patient with severe asthma or reversible airways obstruction in whom regular high doses have been shown to be beneficial
- Prophylactic medication, for example, corticosteroid, to a patient who has difficulty using other inhalational devices
- An antibiotic to a patient with a chronic purulent chest infection (for example, in cystic fibrosis)
- Pentamidine for the prophylaxis and treatment of pneumocystis pneumonia (British Medical Association and Royal Pharmaceutical Society of Great Britain, 2006).

PROCEDURE

- Explain the procedure to the patient and obtain consent
- Prepare the equipment
- Check the patient's prescription chart following the local administration of medicines policy to ensure that the nebulised drug, for example, salbutamol, has been prescribed and is due
- Check the expiry date of the nebulised solution, for example, salbutamol
- Ensure the patient is in a comfortable position, as upright as possible. This may be in a chair or, if the patient is acutely ill, in a bed
- If a nebulised bronchodilator is being administered, it is standard practice to obtain a pre (and post) administration peak expiratory flow (PEF) reading
- Place the compressor on a suitable surface near the patient and plug it into the mains. Clean following local infection control policy and ensure the filter is in place
- Assemble the nebuliser (mask or mouthpiece) as appropriate. It is usual practice to label and retain the packaging as this can be used to store the nebuliser when not in use (Porter-Jones, 2000a)
- Connect the tubing between the nebuliser and the compressor
- Prepare the nebuliser: unscrew the top and pour the prescribed nebulised solution into the nebuliser chamber
- Ensure the top is firmly re-applied to the nebuliser chamber
- Turn on the compressor; the solution to be nebulised should start to 'mist'
- Assist the patient to apply the mask or mouthpiece
- Remind the patient that it is important to breathe through their mouth and not to talk during the procedure (Porter-Jones, 2000b)
- Ask the patient to tap on the nebuliser chamber every few minutes – this will help to prevent condensation developing
- Once 'misting' has stopped, switch off the compressor and remove the mask or mouthpiece. There is usually a small residual volume of nebulised solution at the bottom of the chamber
- Wash and dry the nebuliser chamber following local infection control guidelines and place pack in package for storage
- Offer the patient a drink following the procedure

- Document that the nebuliser has been administered following local protocols
- In some hospitals it is usual practice to repeat the measurement of PEF
- Wash and dry hands
- NB it is usual practice for acutely ill patients to receive their nebuliser using an oxygen supply: connect the nebuliser tubing from the oxygen flow meter to the nebuliser chamber and set the oxygen flow rate to 6–8 litres per minute unless instructed otherwise (Porter-Jones, 2000b).

USE OF A NON-REBREATHE OXYGEN MASK

INTRODUCTION

The non-rebreathe oxygen mask enables the delivery of high concentrations of oxygen and is recommended for use in critically ill patients, ideally guided by pulse oximetry (Resuscitation Council UK, 2011). To ensure the mask is functioning correctly and is effectively used, the manufacturer recommends simple basic checks prior to use (Intersurgical, 2003).

DESCRIPTION

The non-rebreathe oxygen mask (sometimes called a Hudson mask) with an oxygen reservoir bag can be used to deliver high concentrations of oxygen to a spontaneously breathing patient (Jevon, 2007b) (see Figure 12.2 for an image of a non-rebreathing mask). A one-way valve diverts the oxygen flow into the reservoir bag during expiration; the contents of the reservoir bag, together with the high flow oxygen, results in minimal entrainment of air and an inspired oxygen concentration of approximately 85% (Gwinnutt, 2006). The valve also prevents the patient's exhaled gases from contaminating the reservoir bag. The use of the oxygen reservoir bag helps to increase the inspired oxygen concentration by preventing oxygen loss during inspiration (Jevon, 2007b).

It is important to select a sufficient oxygen flow rate to ensure the oxygen reservoir bag does not collapse during inspiration (Resuscitation Council UK, 2011). An oxygen flow rate of 12–15 litres/minute is recommended (Gwinnutt, 2006). Some non-rebreathe masks have elasticated earloop bands, thus eliminating the need to move the patient's head; these are usually used in accident and emergency departments for trauma patients (Jevon, 2007b).

PROCEDURE

- Ensure the patient is upright (to maximise breathing)
- Attach pulse oximetry

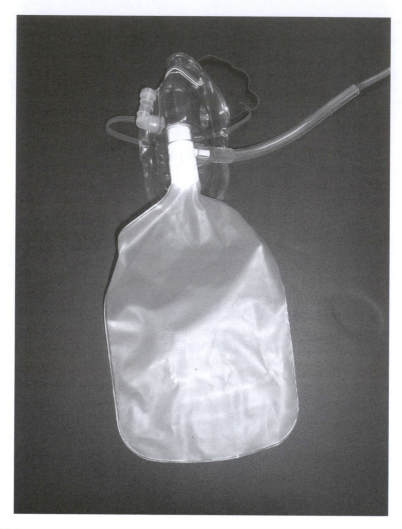

Figure 12.2

- Check the oxygen prescription and explain the procedure to the patient
- Attach the oxygen tubing to the oxygen source and select an oxygen flow rate of 12–15 litres/min (Gwinnutt, 2006)
- Occlude the valve between the mask and the oxygen reservoir bag and check that the reservoir bag is filling up. Remove the finger
- Squeeze the oxygen reservoir bag to check the patency of the valve between the mask and the reservoir bag. If the valve is working correctly it will be possible to empty the reservoir bag (if the reservoir bag does not empty, discard it and select another mask (Smith, 2003)

- Again occlude the valve between the mask and the oxygen reservoir bag allowing the reservoir bag to fill up
- Place the mask with a filled oxygen reservoir bag on the patient's face, ensuring a snug fit
- Reassure the patient
- Closely monitor the patient's vital signs. In particular, assess the patient's response to the oxygen therapy, for example: respiratory rate, mechanics of breathing, colour, oxygen saturation levels, level of consciousness. It may be necessary to monitor arterial blood gases
- Discontinue/reduce the inspired oxygen concentration as appropriate, following advice from a suitably qualified practitioner
- Document the procedure following local protocols (Higgins, 2005) (*Sources*: Intersurgical, 2003; Jevon, 2007b).

RESPIRATORY RATE INDICATOR

Some masks have a respiratory rate indicator to help the healthcare practitioner to monitor the patient's respiratory rate. This indicator can be affected by:

- The patient's respiratory rate
- The orientation of the indicator
- The oxygen flow rate
- The fit of the mask to the patient's face
- The presence of moisture in the indicator tube – which can actually stop the indicator from working (Intersurgical, 2003).

It is important to remember that the respiratory rate indicator should be used as a guide only to monitoring the patient's breathing.

PRESCRIPTION OF OXYGEN THERAPY

Oxygen is a drug and should be prescribed by an appropriately qualified practitioner. This prescription should include:

- Type of oxygen delivery system
- Percentage of oxygen to be delivered (or flow rate)
- Duration of oxygen therapy
- Monitoring that will need to be undertaken (Smith, 2003).

Nursing and Midwifery guidelines for the administration of medications (NMC, 2004) and British National Forumulary guidelines (BMA and RPS, 2010) should be followed. However, in the emergency situation oxygen may need to be administered following local protocols.

PULSE OXIMETRY

INTRODUCTION

Pulse oximetry is a simple non-invasive method of monitoring the percentage of the oxygenation of a patient's haemoglobin (Hb). The pulse oximeter consists of a probe which is attached to a patient's finger, ear lobe or toe. It displays the oxygen saturation and has an audible signal for each pulse beat.

A source of light originates from the probe at two wavelengths and can pick up the saturated haemoglobin; it can then work out the percentage of saturated oxygen.

The oximeter is dependant on pulsatile flow and, therefore, such equipment should be used by appropriately trained people as there are a variety of reasons why a false reading can be obtained. It should be used as a guide to a patient's status and advice should be sought if the healthcare professional is in any doubt.

BACKGROUND

The first pulse oximeter was designed in 1935 and was an ear probe; it developed over the years and in 1987 was first used in theatres to monitor surgical patients.

In 2009, the technology that primary care trusts are now using – Telehealth – had been developed. It is installed in patients' homes and monitors vital signs including pulse oximetry; the information is then transferred by Bluetooth to an appropriate healthcare professional.

There are certain points to remember when performing the skill:

- It provides no guidance on the levels of CO_2, therefore has an important limitation in the care of the respiratory patient
- A reduction in the peripheral pulsatile blood flow (for example, hypovolaemia, severe hypotension, cold ambient temperature, some cardiac arrhythmias such as atrial fibrillation, and peripheral vascular disease), may lead to an inadequate signal and give a false result
- Poor positioning of the probe can cause an altered reading
- Bright overhead lights, as in theatre, can alter the reading
- Shivering/rigor can affect a reading
- In surgery, if methylene blue is used for parathyroid localisation, a short-lived reduction in saturations can occur
- Nail varnish can cause false readings, although jaundice, dark skin or anaemia does not affect the reading.

GETTING READY TO PERFORM THE SKILL

- The healthcare professional will need to introduce themselves and explain to the patient what they intend to do

- The healthcare professional will need a pulse oximeter
- Verbal consent should be obtained prior to commencement
- The patient should be in a comfortable position
- The healthcare professional should assess the patient for any of the adverse reading affects that could occur throughout the skill.

STEP-BY-STEP APPROACH – PROCEDURE

- The patient's hand should be resting on the chest at the level of the heart. The digit used should not be in the air in order to minimise motion artefact. The digit on the arm which is also having a blood pressure done should not be used at the same time as a low reading will occur
- Once the probe is on the digit the healthcare professional should ensure that the light from the oximeter is working
- Ensure that a pulse reading is visible and that a saturation reading is recording
- Wait at least one minute to ensure an accurate reading

All readings should be documented accurately and if the patient is on oxygen, this needs to be charted and the correct litres per minute listed.

CONCLUSION

Pulse oximetry has an important role in the care of all patients, whether in hospital or at home. It does not replace arterial blood gas analysis, as pulse oximetry only measures peripheral oxygenation.

The patient should be fully assessed as to the accuracy of the reading and the healthcare professional needs to be aware of the importance of holistic assessment and the clinical appearance of the patient.

Respiratory Skills

All the respiratory skills described above can be taught using a standard asthmatic patient scenario.

Introduction to Simulation/Scenario

The 'patient' is a 30-year-old asthmatic who is admitted with an acute asthma attack.

Learning Objectives

- Demonstrate ABCDE assessment of the critically ill asthmatic patient
- Demonstrate safe use of oxygen
- Demonstrate correct technique for PEF
- Demonstrate correct technique for use of an inhaler and space device

SIMULATION SCENARIO

- Demonstrate correct technique for pulse oximetry
- Demonstrate correct technique for using a nebuliser.

Resources

Equipment

Appropriate human patient simulator manikin, oxygen source and mask, PEF meter, Ventolin inhaler, spacer device, nebuliser, observation chart, ECG monitor, pulse oximeter, sputum pot with 'green sputum', EWS chart, BTS asthma guidelines, patient's prescription chart

Situation/Scenario

Set up manikin (mild asthma); initial settings:

- RR 28
- Heart rate 90
- BP – 130/80
- Bilateral wheeze
- Oxygen sats – 92% (air), 96% (oxygen)
- Sputum pot – green sputum (chest infection)
- Talking clearly
- Patient lying down in bed.

After sitting patient up, PEF and Ventolin inhaler and oxygen, patient starts to deteriorate (severe asthma):

- RR 36
- Heart rate 110
- BP – 145/80
- Bilateral wheeze
- Oxygen sats – 89% (oxygen)
- Sputum pot – green sputum (chest infection)
- Talking – incomplete sentences
- EWS – call for immediate help, nebuliser

Roles of Participants (if Required) with an Explanation of their Task

Lead participant – to assess and reassess, following the ABCDE approach.

Areas for Discussion and Debrief Technique, if Applicable

- Importance of ABCDE approach
- Importance of following British Thoracic Society (BTS) guidelines.

REFERENCES

Asthma UK (2007) Spacers. Availabe on: www.asthma.org.uk/all_about_asthma/medicines_ treatments/ spacers.html (accessed 29 March 2011).

British Medical Association and Royal Pharmaceutical Society of Great Britain (BMA and RPS) (2006) *British National Formulary*. London: BMJ Publishing.

British Medical Association and Royal Pharmaceutical Society of Great Britain (BMA and RPS) (2010) *British National Formulary*. London: BMJ Publishing.

British Thoracic Society (BTS) and Scottish Intercollegiate Network (SIGN) (2008) *Update to the British Guideline on the Management of Asthma*. Originally published February 2003. Available on: www.sign.ac.uk [accessed 29 March 2011].

Currie, G. and Douglas, J. (2007) 'Oxygen and inhalers', in G. Currie (ed.), *ABC of COPD*. Oxford: Blackwell Publishing, Oxford, pp. 22–4.

Gwinnutt, C. (2006) *Clinical Anaesthesia,* 2nd edn. Oxford: Blackwell Publishing.

Hardwell, A., Barber, V., Hargadon, T., McKnight, E., Holmes, J. and Levy, M.L. (2009) 'Technique training does not improve the ability of most patients to use pressured metered dose inhalers', *Primary Care Respiratory Journal*, 20 (1): 92–6.

Higgins, D. (2005) 'Oxygen therapy', *Nursing Times*, 101 (4): 30–1.

Intersurgical (2003) *Non-rebreathing Mask Product Literature*. Wokingham: Intersurgical.

Jevon, P. (2007a) 'Respiratory procedures: use of a nebuliser', *Nursing Times*, 103 (34): 24–5.

Jevon, P. (2007b) 'Respiratory procedures: use of a non-rebreathing oxygen mask', *Nursing Times*, 103 (32): 26–7.

Nursing and Midwifery Council (NMC) (2004) *Guidelines for the Administration of Medicines*. London: NMC.

O'Callaghan, C. and Barry, P. (1997) 'The science of nebulised drug delivery', *Thorax*, 52 (Suppl 2): S31–S44 S31.

Pearce, L. (2000) 'KNOW HOW Inhaler devices', *Nursing Times*, 96 (37): 16.

Porter-Jones, G. (2000a) 'Nebulisers – 1: Preparation', *Nursing Times,* 96 (36): 45–6.

Porter-Jones, G. (2000b) 'Nebulisers – 2: Administration', *Nursing Times,* 96 (37): 51–2.

Rees, J. and Kanabar, D. (2006) *ABC of Asthma,* 5th edn. Oxford: Blackwell.

Resuscitation Council UK (2011) *Advanced life Support*, 6th edn. London: Resuscitation Council (UK).

Smith, G. (2003) *ALERT*, 2nd edn. Portsmouth: University of Portsmouth.

13

DEALING WITH MENTAL HEALTH EMERGENCIES

Simon Steeves

Aim

The aim of this chapter is to give an overview of common mental health issues and basic assessment and management strategies of how to deal with them.

Objectives

The learning objectives for this chapter are for the learner to be able to:

- Recognise the symptoms of common mental health (MH) problems – the learner will understand the symptoms of MH illnesses and be able to assess the mental state of the person while respecting that person, recognising the importance of the individual's experience and promoting person-centred and recovery-based practice (NMC standards for pre-registration education in mental health nursing 4.1, 2010)
- Predict the likelihood of and deal with MH emergencies – to demonstrate an understanding of patterns which indicate an increase in the severity of a condition and may lead to an emergency
- Develop good practice in a safe environment – using simulation will promote good practice that addresses potential power imbalances between professionals and people experiencing mental health problems, including situations where compulsory measures are used (NMC standards for pre-registration education in mental health nursing 2.1, 2010). There are times in mental health nursing when interventions carry some risk. Being able to experience positive risk-taking in the classroom will support students when faced with issues in practice. Sometimes we must consider that just because we can do something it

is not implicit that we should. It must also be considered that the way we do things will not always be identical but change according to circumstances. The ethical implications of our interventions will always be considered before action is taken

- Develop understanding of current legislation – mental health nurses must understand and apply current legislation to all service users, especially in emergencies (NMC standards for pre-registration education in mental health nursing 1.1, 2010)

The NMC code of conduct outlines all these competencies as being achieved in order for anyone to attain registration and practice as a mental health nurse.

INTRODUCTION

Any discussions on mental health (MH) issues are, by their very nature, complex. MH problems are superimposed on an existing personality. This means that, as we are all unique individuals, the presentation of a condition will never be exactly the same in any two individuals. For example, a broken leg will follow the same care pathway – reduction, immobilising or possibly surgical repair – in all people regardless of gender, race, culture or creed. However, a diagnosis in MH will not predetermine the behaviours or presentation in all people.

MH emergencies will almost exclusively be dealt with by MH nurses; doctors may prescribe medication or oversee seclusion, but they are unlikely to be involved in de-escalation or restraint. For this reason this chapter will refer to the Nursing and Midwifery Council's competencies for nurses in order to highlight some of the necessary components to this care. This does not mean that the chapter is only aimed at nurses but to demonstrate the areas for discussion and explain why they are necessary. Inevitably there will be circumstances where anyone may have to deal with a person with MH issues. Incidents may happen anywhere, so even a member of the public with no training may be involved. With this in mind, this chapter will look at aggressive or disinhibited behaviours and try to give some guidelines for dealing with these behaviours or preventing them.

The Nursing and Midwifery Council (NMC) standards for pre-registration education in mental health nursing clearly specify knowledge of legislation (competency 1.1) and power imbalances between the professional and the person experiencing mental health problems (competency 2.1). These competencies are noted in the Learning Objectives.

Obviously all nurses and health professionals need to be aware of the law, for example, consent and capacity to consent, but in mental health nursing the law carries far greater impact. The Mental Health Act 2007 impacts on almost all aspects of care in mental health nursing. Not only must the Mental Health Act Code of Practice be followed, but it must also be used in conjunction with the Mental Health Capacity Act 2005 (now embedded in the Mental Health Act 2007) and also with the Deprivation of Liberty Safeguards. It is not our intention to produce a book on law in detail so we address these issues only where relevant in further sections in this chapter.

The power imbalances between professionals and those experiencing mental health problems must also be considered far more intently in mental health and learning disability than other branches of healthcare. Historically there is a perception that this client group is incapable of helping themselves and that they rely on professionals to tell them what to do and how to behave; 'the historical dominance of the medical model of "mental illness" underpins the popular conception of mentally distressed individuals as irrational and dependent on the intervention of others' (Coppock and Hopton, 2000: 157). In adult branch nursing most of the clients are willing participants in their care with a shared objective of becoming well again. Emergencies in mental health nursing cross the boundaries between branches. As stated by Clarke and Walsh, 'An understanding of the structure and function of the human body should be central to the education of all health professionals' (Clarke and Walsh, 2009: 10). For example, mental health nurses will meet physical conditions such as respiratory collapse in drug overdose, convulsions and seizures in alcohol withdrawal, and obesity and its associated problems in severe enduring mental health. However, one of the main issues can be challenging behaviour in patients suffering from perceptual impairment disorders. Without wishing to highlight violence and aggression as a main symptom of mental health nursing, it exists and is therefore a valid area to explore. Warren, cited in the Sainsbury Report, states that 'Incidents involving violence are reported to be on the increase' (Sainsbury Centre for Mental Health, 1998). Many of the learners will not have faced irrational aggression before and so simulation is probably a better and safer way to explore it.

It is hoped in this chapter to set clear learning objectives, give an example of a scenario, and discuss the work that learners will undertake, as well as the other considerations necessary for successful completion of this work. There will be an example of a scenario that will support the achievement of the necessary competencies to be achieved.

UNDERSTANDING MENTAL HEALTH PROBLEMS, RECOGNIZING INCREASED RISK AND DEALING WITH CRISIS

A mental health problem that is moving into crisis and is in danger of becoming an emergency is normally measured by risk to self or others. It is not the intention of this chapter to describe all mental health problems in detail so a brief overview is offered, describing some of the symptoms, how the learner will recognise an increase in severity, and how to measure risk and manage the crisis before it becomes an emergency.

Mental health problems are clearly defined in the Diagnostic and Statistical Manual of Mental Disorders 4 (DSM 4) (American Psychiatric Association, 2000) and the International Classification of Diseases 10 (ICD10) (World Health Organization, 1992) but for the purpose of this discussion it is simpler to look at only three general categories: psychotic, affective and behavioural. Psychotic problems include perceptual impairment illnesses such as schizophrenia, drug-induced psychosis and some physical conditions which can cause psychotic phenomena. Affective problems include the mood disorders of which the most common are bi-polar affective disorder, hypomania and depression. The behavioural problems may include self harm, binge drinking, aggression and violence. This group is not without contention as the 'mad or bad' debate centres heavily around behavioural problems. The murky hinterland between madness and badness pervades the conceptualisation of mental illness. (Elder and Holmes, 2002).

PSYCHOTIC PROBLEMS

PSYCHOTIC PROBLEMS – THE MAIN SYMPTOMS

In psychotic problems the symptoms fall into three main categories: hallucinations, delusions and lifestyle changes.

Hallucinations are defined as 'sensory perception in the absence of sensor stimuli' (Clarke and Walsh, 2009: 184). Hallucinations can affect all of the five senses, for example, 'hearing voices' is an auditory experience of someone talking to you when no one is present. In cases of severe withdrawal from alcohol the person may feel insects crawling over their skin – tactile hallucinations. The other three hallucinations are referred to as visual, olfactory (smell) and gustatory (taste).

Delusions are defined as 'being a false and fixed idea that does not correspond to the person's usual belief system and is held despite evidence to the contrary' (Clarke and Walsh, 2009: 280). An example of this may be where the person has a religious delusion where they believe themselves to be a deity or the child of a deity.

Lifestyle changes may be the result of delusions or what is known as negative symptoms. The negative symptoms of schizophrenia include emotional withdrawal, avolition (passive, apathetic, social withdrawal) and a dysfunctional relationship with others (Shives, 2008).

PSYCHOTIC PROBLEMS – ASSESSING INCREASED RISK

A person may not always be seen to be hallucinating so the learner needs to develop their observational skills. Apart from the more obvious symptoms, where the person may be shouting at others who are not there, signs of increased MH problems may include:

- Increased level of distraction, for example, an inability to concentrate or answer a question
- Increase in non-compliance, for example, the refusal of regular medication
- Increased levels of agitation, constant pacing or wanting to leave the area without giving a reason
- Increased level of withdrawal, spending long hours alone in their room or long hours listening through headphones
- Increased levels of previous known behaviours, for example, exhibiting a pattern of behaviour which has previously resulted in violence or aggression.

DEALING WITH THE CRISIS

The most important issue in dealing with the crisis is to assess risk. The new MH nurse or any other person must prioritise personal safety. If the symptoms exhibited are inducing fears, then always raise the alarm and leave if you can. Any professional MH nurse would rather attend several false alarms than one tragedy.

Risk may be assessed by:

- Agitation, pacing, aggressive behaviours – thumping walls or other violent demonstrative behaviour
- Raised voices, shouting, foul language or abuse of the learner – violent abuse, sexual abuse, racial abuse or any abuse which de-personalises the learner. De-personalisation is the process whereby the identity of a person is removed, to allow harm to befall them without guilt. For example, during the Vietnam War, American troops did not want to shoot fathers, brothers, wives or children so they referred to the Vietnamese people as Gooks, Charlie or Kong
- Body language which suggests violence – clenched fists, exaggerated movements of the hands or feet, or sudden movements towards another person
- An apparent disregard for personal space – what some people refer to as 'getting in your face'.

Having assessed the risk:

- Decide whether you have the skills to cope with this level of risk. There is no shame in choosing to raise the alarm. As Shakespeare's character Falstaff remarked 'The better part of valor is discretion, in the which better part I have sav'd my life.'
- What is your relationship to this client? Do you have what could be called a 'therapeutic relationship' or have you only just met them? How well you know them will affect their ability to de-personalise
- Consider the environment, look for your nearest exit route and do not allow anyone to block it
- Try to talk quietly and calmly to the client
- Assess their responses; are they calmer or the same in tone?
- Constantly reassess and introduce yourself to maintain personal contact
- If the client is merely damaging property, is intervention necessary?
- Should a form of restraint become necessary, always use the least force necessary, ensure the safety of all especially the client, have regard for the dignity of the client and protect other clients who may witness the event. The Mental Health Act Code of Practice (1983 amended 1999) gives an excellent overview of patients presenting particular management problems in chapter 19, which is essential reading to inform the discussion above (MHA Code of Practice, 1983/1999). More detail is provided in further reading at the end of this chapter.

AFFECTIVE PROBLEMS

AFFECTIVE PROBLEMS – THE MAIN SYMPTOMS

Although mood disorders, previously referred to as affective problems (Shives, 2008), present as elation or depression, in extreme levels these may shift into psychosis. People who suffer from bi-polar affective disorder may become psychotic and exhibit strong delusional states, often extremely grandiose. Therefore, in this part of the chapter we will discuss only the less extreme symptoms as the more extreme are detailed above within the discussion of psychotic problems. These symptoms include:

- Changes in lifestyle including lack of interest in pursuits previously enjoyed, withdrawal from society, or poor self care; loss of appetite, sleeplessness, poor concentration
- Mood affected more than usual – a song or film making the person cry more than usual
- Lability of mood – one minute laughing and the next minute angry or crying
- Increasing low mood, crying continually
- Feelings of hopelessness or worthlessness
- Thoughts of suicide.

AFFECTIVE PROBLEMS – ASSESSING INCREASED RISK

When people become depressed they may suffer loss of interest and enjoyment, becoming isolated and alone. 'Many if not most of the clinical features of depression are present to such an intense degree that the patient finds it difficult to fulfil his or her social obligations' (Burton, 2006: 65). This increases the risk of their low mood going unnoticed. The same can be said of those who are beginning to demonstrate elated behaviour; they may appear happy, carefree and enjoying themselves. Factors increasing the risk in high or low mood are:

- Not attending work or social functions, especially those they have usually enjoyed
- Becoming less contactable, not answering the phone or messages
- Changes in appearance, these changes can be either the client becoming less well dressed or, in elevated mood, increasingly flamboyant
- Disinhibited behaviour; risky behaviour
- Increase in lability of mood, especially tearfulness to anger
- Writing of letters predicting their death, wills or disposal of property
- Secreting or storing medication, especially those medications known to kill such as paracetamol
- Suicidal ideation or the expression of a wish to die.

DEALING WITH THE CRISIS

As with functional problems, risk assessment is a priority. The risk factors we have already discussed in the assessment need to be the result of observation. Observation in MH has been a source of complaint for many clients. Observation does not just mean watching someone; it means talking to them, observing body language and noting changes from the last time you spoke.

If someone expresses suicidal ideation, the learner must explore the risk. The risk increases as the questions in the following list are answered with a yes:

- Does the client express a wish to die?
- Have they decided on a plan or method?
- Have they taken action – bought pills or a hose pipe for instance?
- Do they have a time frame?

If all these questions gain a 'yes' response then this client is at extreme risk of suicide.

In more elated mood, the observer needs to look out for increases in risky behaviours and the possible development of psychotic phenomena. If the early onset of these is noted, then early intervention with medication and nursing care to protect them from risk and harm are paramount.

BEHAVIOURAL DISORDERS

The symptoms associated with behavioural disorders will be similar to affective disorders. There is much debate about diagnoses such as personality disorder, but it is irrelevant to this chapter. The risks, assessment process and care is much the same as for any person who is distressed by their mental health problem.

BACKGROUND TO THE SKILL

As children we learn by observation, imitation and repetition to develop our life skills. Jean Piaget, the swiss developmental psychologist, saw children as actively constructing their own development, through their interactions with the environment. The importance of direct activity holds true for the young infant as much as for the older child (Davis, 1994). Simulation offers the same opportunities to students. The skills of the experienced practitioner can be demonstrated and seen by the student who can then imitate, have repeated attempts, and learn correct and safe practice.

Experienced practitioners in mental health very often refer to having had 'a gut feeling' about an event or prediction of an event. It can be argued that this expression sells their skills short. Inevitably it is their knowledge, skill and previous experience which allow them to come to conclusions about these events. When they have been part of the care for many types of illness and seen many people treated successfully, practitioners build up an extensive knowledge base from which to draw. A successful educator can provide prior experience of events to their students using simulation.

Dealing with challenging behaviour carries a high level of risk. The skills of remaining calm and supportive when faced with aggression can be safely learned in the classroom, with the support of a competent facilitator, and hopefully when things go wrong they can be addressed without harm to the participants.

GETTING READY TO PERFORM THE SKILL

The resources required for this simulation are few. In terms of equipment there is little required for an interpersonal experience working with people. The scenario would need to be printed out for the students, possibly laminated for future use, or provided as an overhead projection which could remain up for the duration of the exercise. When using simulation, students report that they prefer their own written copy, allowing them to write notes on it and use it as reference. The tutor might also need to consider a set of cards for each group, giving out the roles. Students will invariably challenge for roles they either want or want to avoid. Gender should not be considered in allocating roles as it can be of great value to experience how others see the experience and what factors are affected by gender.

The setting needs to be comfortable and spacious. When working with small groups in one room there must be space for the students to converse without impinging on others' conversations. It is ideal to have the room set up before the students arrive. As the scenario is set in a bedroom, the use of beds and screens, if possible, may help to enhance the realistic feeling of the action.

The time element needs to be well balanced. If there is too much time, discussion can often move from the task in hand and lose focus altogether. Conversely, if too little time is allocated the student may feel that the exercise has been trivialised. About one hour would seem appropriate. The learning experience can be improved by giving a break after this and then getting the whole group to share their discussions and thinking.

It must be considered that in any group work using role-play, it is the responsibility of the facilitator to ensure student safety. It is important that you notice if a student becomes distressed. For this purpose it is important to limit the size of the group to a manageable level. When working in groups, if a group exceeds 10 participants it might be necessary to use a 'lifeguard'. This person does not join in the activity but simply observes and is able to flag up any potential problems before or as they arise. It might be useful to replicate this role when working with large groups.

Prior to starting the simulation it might be useful to discuss the use of foul language and abuse. Nurses in mental health will suffer abuse but they must understand that it is not about them but about the disempowerment of the clients they meet and the power exchange. Discussion could also help learners to understand about the types of abuse they may suffer. The power exchange relies on the effect of abuse. Accordingly the abuser will seek to touch on areas that have most effect: students from black and ethnic minority groups will face racial abuse, young females may suffer sexual abuse, and those who are larger may face fattist abuse (NMC code of conduct 2.1, 2008).

PROCEDURE

Scenarios for close to real-life practice have been developed and used for some time. In the book, *Gamesters' Handbook*, it is noted that 'Games generate interest: they need enthusiasm. Used with purpose they can be the framework upon which all other work is developed' (Brandes and Phillips, 1977: 984). This scenario takes place on an Acute Mental Health ward at breakfast time.

Table 13.1

Activities	Process
The scenario will take place as a role-play	Consider a set of cards for each group giving out the roles. Alternatively, given the effect of some roles, it may be advisable to allow the students to discuss them beforehand
Learners will role-play the roles opposite	The roles to be played out are: • A young female client who is refusing medication and displaying sexually disinhibited behaviour • A young man with a diagnosis of schizophrenia who has in the past demonstrated aggressive behaviour • One trained nurse • Four care assistants
A care assistant finds the two clients in bed in the young man's room	Consider what action the care assistant should take
The young man becomes very angry and abusive claiming that he and the young woman are in a relationship	When the other staff arrive what attitudes and manner should they adopt?

AREAS FOR DISCUSSION

As previously stated in the introduction and learning outcomes, there are three main areas for discussion by the students: clinical, legal and ethical considerations. These will be outlined as separate categories.

Clinical considerations: When looking at the scenario, students will be expected to discuss the delivery of care to the clients. How are they going to deal with the situation maintaining the safety of all involved and protecting the clients from actions which might be deemed irrational? Person-centred care requires the client to be placed at the centre of care. To deny someone their right to choose returns care to the medical model in which the professional (expert) and the client (dependent) strengthen the power imbalance between the two.

The young man is expecting to go to the General Hospital today for an outpatient appointment, having complained of back pain for some time. The students may also consider cancelling the outpatient visit, but will have to weigh up the impact this will have on the client. How long has he been waiting for this? What is the client's expected outcome? Is he in pain? All these factors will have to be taken into consideration. It is well known that pain is individual to the person suffering it and that chronic pain is one of the risk factors in suicide (National Pain Foundation, 2011). A decision needs to be reached on the young woman refusing medication. We obviously have a duty of care here but this might require some element of restraint. This decision will also be dealt with in both of the following areas.

Legal considerations: The normally open ward is locked for management reasons. All current legislation – that is, the Mental Health Act and the Mental Capacity Act – state that clients must be treated in the least restrictive manner. Locking the door to protect one or two clients impacts directly on the rights of the others. What do the learners propose as an action plan for addressing this issue? The young woman is of an age to consent to sex but does she have the capacity? How would the students assess her capacity under the law? What are the client's rights in this case? The students will also have to consider the legal right to give medication, including the use of restraint, and the method they will use.

Ethical considerations: As stated above the nurses have the legal authority to administer medication using restraint. The students will need to consider how to do this in an ethical manner. There are five staff members on duty but only three are female. The nurses who will be involved in this interaction will have to be chosen carefully. The students will have to consider the effect on this young woman of their actions. What would be the effect on this vulnerable young woman to be restrained by men, be exposed to them and then injected? What action could the team take to minimise her distress? It is possible that the participants may need to develop assertive skills to negotiate on behalf of the client. In her book on asserting yourself, Keenan states 'When you accept that you have rights and that others do too, it is easier to realise when those rights are being infringed' (Keenan, 1999: 108). Using simulation can develop the understanding of assertiveness and develop the skill of being so. The very fact of giving roles can allow people a voice that they may otherwise not feel they have.

The learners will have to practise the skills necessary for de-escalating the situation and use both verbal and non-verbal techniques. These techniques hold some basic rules.

When responding to violence and aggression nurses should:

- Remain calm
- Speak slowly and softly
- Consider their stance. A sideways stance is advised as a smaller target is offered and vital organs are less likely to be injured
- Try to keep hands open
- Try to get the aggressor to sit down
- Avoid getting into an argument.

It is also important to be aware of the use of debriefing and supervision at the end of these sessions. In simulation it is sometimes easy to forget that the participants are playing a role and for the person to become emotional about that role. Research has shown that 'relative to equivalent non-NHS organisations, local staff had higher levels of mental and physical ill-health associated with job-related stress' (Duncan-Grant, 2001: 116). The stresses that can arise during role-play can often be taken away from the classroom as baggage and affect the relationships between participants. As stated earlier, the learners can be brought back into a larger group which not only deepens the learning experience but it normalises the activity and brings learners back to their real roles – who they really are – rather than the role they have been playing. It is useful to allow learners to talk about how they felt during simulation rather than solely about what they learnt.

The learners must also be allowed to talk about their emotions and feelings during the role-play. Anyone who has been involved in an aggressive incident will have feelings, possibly fear or anger. These emotions are perfectly valid and need to be discussed. It may be that the facilitator might want to get the group to engage in some light-hearted activity to help feelings to return to normal.

CONCLUSION

The use of simulation is well documented and understood. It is a powerful tool for deep learning and, properly managed, carries little risk. The numbers and types of scenarios are as wide ranging as the people who will be using them. The effect of using scenarios can also improve incidental learning. This is defined in *A Dictionary of Human Behaviour* as 'Learning that takes place without a conscious effort, e.g., learning the names of the shop on the way to the bus stop' (Statt, 1981: 204). The fact of role playing and gaining new experiences can very often teach us things as we go along without us struggling to commit facts to memory. In this simulation the learners can learn a lot about themselves as well as the necessary skills for de-escalation. Finally, working in groups can be an empowering and supportive activity. Although Yalom was writing about therapy in the following quotation, I feel he sums up group working nicely, 'Cohesiveness favors self disclosure, risk taking, and the constructive expression of conflict in the group – phenomena that facilitate successful therapy' (Yalom 1985: 76).

FURTHER READING

The Mental Health Act Code of Practice 1983 amended 1999.
This is now further updated so to find the advice given on managing the difficult patient (Chapter 19) you will need to research. The full reference can be found in the reference list at the end of this chapter.

REFERENCES

American Psychiatric Association (2000) *Diagnostic and Statistical Manual of Mental Disorders IV*. Arlington: American Psychiatric Association.

Brandes, D. and Phillips, H. (1977) *Gamesters' Handbook*. London: Hutchinson.

Burton, N. (2006) *Psychiatry*. Oxford: Blackwell Publishing.

Clarke, V. and Walsh, A. (2009) *Fundamentals of Mental Health Nursing*. Oxford: Oxford University Press.

Coppock, V. and Hopton, J. (2000) *Critical Perspectives on Mental Health*. London: Routledge.

Davis, A. (1994) cited in P. Light, S. Sheldon and M. Woodhead (1994) *Learning to Think*. London: Routledge.

Duncan-Grant, A. (2001) *Clinical Supervision Activity among Mental Health Nurses*. Portsmouth: Nursing Praxis International.

Elder, A. and Holmes, J. (2002) *Mental Health in Primary Care*. Oxford: Oxford University Press.

Keenan, K. (1999) *Management Guide to Asserting Yourself*. London: Oval Books.

Mental Capacity Act (2005) London: HMSO.

Mental Health Act (2007) London: HMSO.

Mental Health Act Code of Practice (1983/1999) London: HMSO.

National Pain Foundation (2011) *Chronic Pain and Suicide Risk*. Available on: http://www.nationalpainfoundation.org/articles/290/chronic-pain-and-suicide-risk [accessed 9 May 2011].

Nursing and Midwifery Council (2008) *The Code: Standards of Conduct, Perfomance and Ethics for Nurses and Midwives*. London: NMC. Available on: http://standards.nmc-uk.org/Pages/Downloads.aspx [accessed 20 June 2011].

Sainsbury Centre for Mental Health (1998) *Acute Problems*. London: Sainsbury Centre for Mental Health.

Shives, L. (2008) *Basic Concepts of Psychiatric – Mental Health Nursing*. Philadelphia, PA: Lippincot, Williams and Wilkins.

Statt, D. (1981) *A Dictionary of Human Behaviour*. London: Harper & Row.

World Health Organization (1992) *The International Statistical Classification of Diseases and Related Health Problems 10*. Washington: World Health Organization.

Yalom, I. (1985) *The Theory and Practice of Group Psychotherapy*. New York: Basic Books.

14

PRINCIPLES OF PATIENT HANDLING

Steve Wanless

Aim

The aim of this chapter is to give healthcare professionals an insight into and strategies for teaching the importance of correct posture and positioning when performing patient and inanimate load handling. The chapter also aims to make learners aware of the risks associated with patient handling.

Objectives

- To demonstrate the skills required to maintain correct posture and positioning during patient handling activities and facilitate safe movement
- To increase awareness of individual risk assessment and the safe handling of loads
- To reduce the risk of occupational injury while carrying out patient and inanimate load handling tasks.

The contents of this chapter will outline the difference between 'moving and handling principles' and 'techniques'. It is important to understand these differences as they underpin all handling procedures. Moving and handling principles are defined as the safest way for the body to move, while a technique is the key to obtaining certain postures or movements (Health and Safety Executive (HSE), 2003).

Healthcare workers may be shown and taught all the patient handling procedures required for safely handling patients; however, this does not ensure that a safe position will be adopted in order to perform the handling procedure. Without encompassing and using the basic principles of moving and handling, safety will always be compromised. Healthcare workers who follow the principles may injure themselves as the load, being a human being, is an unpredictable load. However, the correct position for handling will help to prevent or minimise any injury.

An estimated one third of all reported injuries in healthcare settings result from moving and handling accidents, while approximately 40 per cent of all sickness absence in the health service is attributed to moving and handling accidents (Department of Health (DH), 2002). It is reported that an estimated 80,000 nurses sustain back injuries at work each year (National Audit Office, 2003). Healthcare professionals exhibit high rates of lower back, neck and shoulder pain that have been attributed to manual patient handling activities (Smedley et al., 2003). Employers are required by law to take reasonable steps to safeguard the health and safety of all their employees, but moving and handling injuries remain disproportionately high.

Safe moving and handling of patients is not just about how the basic principles are applied to patient handling procedures. The principles of patient handling should be incorporated into a safety culture that is implemented from the top level of any organisation that supports and recognises the provision of moving and handling training, and supplying the correct and appropriate level of patient handling equipment. This again should be supported by local management ensuring that safe working practices are being undertaken and assessed appropriately.

INTRODUCTION TO THE SKILL

In Great Britain moving and handling within the workplace is subject to legislation, the implementation of this legislation being supervised through a number of government bodies. Guidance is also available from professional bodies for healthcare practitioners. All the legislation places responsibilities on both the employer and employees with regard to work practice, equipment provision and risk assessment.

There are five main areas of legislation that govern moving and handling at work. These are: the Health and Safety at Work Act 1974, Management of Health and Safety at Work Regulations 1992, Manual Handling Operations Regulations 1992 (Amended), Provision and Use of Work Equipment Regulations 1998, and Lifting Operation and Lifting Equipment Regulations 1998.

HEALTH AND SAFETY AT WORK ACT 1974

This is the enabling Act for all legislation that follows and it sets out minimum requirements for both employers and employees.

The employer is required to provide:

> Such information, instruction, training and supervision as is necessary to ensure, so far as is reasonably practicable, the health and safety at work of his employees.

The Act requires the employee to:

> Take reasonable care for his own safety and the health and safety of other people who may be affected by his or her acts or omissions.

MANUAL HANDLING OPERATIONS REGULATIONS 1992 (AMENDED 2004)

The regulations require the employer to:

- Avoid hazardous manual handling activities as far as is reasonably practicable
- Assess any hazardous manual handling operations that are not avoidable
- Reduce the risk of injury as far as is reasonably practicable
- Review assessments to ensure they are valid, current, suitable and sufficient.

The regulations require employees to:

- Follow the assessed safe system of work and make proper use of equipment provided
- Cooperate with their employers in regards to their health and safety matters
- Advise their manager if they are not fit to carry on with their duties
- Not to put themselves or others at risk of injury by their acts or omissions

A number of professional bodies have also produced written documents in response to the legislation – Royal College of Nursing, Chartered Society of Physiotherapists, Royal College of Midwives and various other bodies. These documents provide practical guidance on moving and handling for their practitioners within the workplace and recommend standards of practice for adoption by the professions as a whole.

All the legislation and the guidance from both statutory and professional bodies recognise that practitioners can contribute to improved safety in their working environment by fulfilling their moving and handling obligations.

There is a significant level of legislation regarding moving and handling for healthcare workers that is supported by statutory and professional body guidance. Healthcare workers are also encouraged to contribute to improving safety in their workplaces and procedures by fulfilling these obligations.

BACKGROUND TO THE SKILL

Healthcare workers are exposed to high levels of patient handling as part of the daily routine. Unlike many other areas, healthcare professionals are required to perform varied practices that include many different facets. The main difference that healthcare workers are subject to is that their manual handling involves human beings rather than just inanimate loads. The handling of a human being does not just constitute overcoming weight but many other factors must be taken into consideration including: the weight, shape and size of the patient; their capability; age; if they will cooperate and other factors that contribute to an increased risk of back injury in this work group (Edlich et al., 2004).

Leggett states that efficient movement of the human body involves the application of principles rather than the learning of techniques (Leggett, 1998). It is also recognised that any training relies upon the correct principles being outlined, understood and applied by the handlers (Health and Safety Executive (HSE), 2003).

An historical culture still remains within the healthcare sector to lift patients manually. Time pressures, expectation from the patient or relatives, lack of equipment, perceived lack of patient cooperation, or other factors are cited that encourage the handler to lift the patient. There has to be an acceptance by not only the handler, but also the employer, that the safety culture has to be recognised and implemented from the top of any organisation. To ensure that members of staff who are required to manually handle patients are working to a safe working practice, the organisation must have a manual handling policy with the roles and responsibilities of all levels of staff contained within it.

Epidemiological studies around the world have consistently identified nursing personnel at high risk of low back pain and musculoskeletal injury (Menzel et al., 2004). The standards set down by Workcover NSW in September 1998 state that 'the approach used in the standards is that safe moving and handling should be based on a set of principles adaptable to a variety of situations' (Workcover, NSW, 1998: 37).

GETTING READY TO PERFORM THE SKILL

The principles of patient handling do not start when you are about to perform a moving and handling procedure with the patient. They begin with the safety culture of the workplace and how the employer provides for a safe working environment. Without this foundation, there will always be a risk of a healthcare worker performing a procedure either without the correct or sufficient equipment or without the sufficient numbers of staff needed to move the patient safely. Healthcare workers may perform an unsafe procedure due to the caring nature of the profession, consequently any patient in discomfort requires intervention.

It is important to note that a caring nature often overrides the need to look after yourself. The one person that is forgotten in this situation is the handler alongside the possible consequences of sustaining a back injury which will not only affect themselves but also their families. The caring health worker may find it difficult to comply with correct moving and handling principles when they appear to counteract the care of the patient. Insufficient staff and time constraints may be used as a reason for not using correct principles; however, the application of a correct principle or principles should not take any longer than performing an incorrect or controversial moving and handling procedure (Health and Safety Executive (HSE), 2003). Safe working practice within any organisation must be contained in a moving and handling policy where the roles and responsibilities of all levels of staff are outlined, reviewed and implemented.

PROCEDURE

There are specific issues relating to the handling of patients which bring forward certain concerns. Examples of areas of concern include: static handling of patients' limbs while being prepared for surgery, handling patients where there may be a need for restraints, characteristics other than the patient's condition, for example, friable skin, osteoporosis, fractures, reflexes or emergency situations.

The individual handler's principles of patient handling start prior to the procedure by the undertaking of a personal risk assessment. Patient handling demands a blend of common sense and being adaptable to any unusual situations that may arise. Due to the fact that the load to be moved is unpredictable, every patient handling task is unique – no two patients are the same and a patient's condition does not stay the same indefinitely. Circumstances can change within a very short time, therefore, it is necessary to stop and conduct a personal risk assessment prior to each moving and handling procedure. The principles of safe patient handling start with a personal risk assessment and the question: 'stop and think, is there a reason for handling or am I performing the task without a correct reason for moving the patient?'. Remember, every time you place your hands on a patient to assist or transfer them, you are at risk of injury.

The overall aim and objective of any patient handling task should always be the first consideration. A moving and handling procedure should only be carried out if there is no other way to achieve the objective, this will help to ensure that the carer will not be caught unprepared or put themselves at risk.

Once it has been accepted that there is a clear objective then a personal risk assessment should be conducted which takes into consideration the following areas: the environment, load, individual capability, the task, and the equipment that is required to perform the manual handling safely. On completion of the assessment the question that needs to be answered is 'Can I or we perform this procedure safely? – Yes or No?'

The answer to this question should be honest; if it is not honest then there is a risk of injury not only to the handler but to colleagues and to the patient. If the answer is positive then the procedure should be acceptable; if, however, the answer is negative then help and advice should be sought. Following advice support, reappraisal of the original assessment should be undertaken and the question asked again.

The questions that should be considered about each area, using the acronym **TILE** (Task, Individual capability, Load, Environment) to ensure a safe outcome to the patient handling procedure, include those listed in Table 14.1.

Table 14.1

Task and what it involves	Does this task need to be undertaken or can it be avoided? Are there any restrictions regarding posture? Does the load need to be held away from the trunk? Is there a long carrying distance? How many times will this procedure be performed and over what period of time? Does it involve any pushing or pulling? Is there a need for prolonged physical effort? Is the task physically or mentally demanding?
Individual capability of handler and colleagues	Is everyone physically fit? Are there any medical or physical conditions that may affect ability? Are there any height constraints or age constraints? Have all parties been trained in that technique or on the equipment? Does clothing hinder movement or posture? Is there any special strength required to perform the task?
Load – the patient	Assess their capability, their weight shape and size. Are they difficult to get hold of? Are they easily managed both physically and mentally? Are they an unbalanced or an unstable load? Are they awkward? Do we need special information about the load, the patient's position and the patient's clothing? Encourage the patient to contribute to each stage of the procedure
Environment	Are there space constraints, slippery floors or different flooring, furniture, cluttered areas, blocked passageways, poor lighting, doors with keypads and swipe cards? Are there issues regarding going up and down stairs, slopes, high or low temperatures and weather conditions? The questions regarding moving and handling equipment – e.g. is the equipment correct for the procedure, is the equipment in safe working order, has the equipment been inspected, what is the safe working load – will run through all of the assessment and not come under one specific area. Good housekeeping of the environment by simple arranging of the handling environment can eliminate slipping or tripping hazards and ensure adequate space and a safe environment

When working with colleagues, in order to ensure that all of the above is taken into consideration, it is necessary to recognise a team leader whose role will be to plan the procedure and give clear and concise instructions. Communicating with colleagues and the patient is paramount to ensure a safe procedure.

Communicating and preparing is the role of the team leader. A full explanation of the procedure should be discussed with the patient in order to encourage the patient to assist if they are able to do so. However, handlers are in charge of the movement. If the patient decides to do their own movement then a full explanation must be repeated – a patient should never be allowed to take charge of an assisted movement. Once the patient is prepared, the handlers then prepare the equipment and the environment, carefully removing all hazards both in the handling area and also along the route taken if transferring a patient. If time has elapsed and the patient may have forgotten the first explanation, another explanation of what will happen and what is expected of the patient should be undertaken.

Once all of the above has been undertaken the handlers must concentrate on position and posture for the procedure. There are several factors that need to be considered in order to reduce the risk of personal injury.

CONTROLLING CENTRE OF GRAVITY BY MAINTAINING A NATURAL BODY ALIGNMENT

Natural Body Alignment is the body's natural position fully supported by the core muscle system from which all movement begins and ends. Side views of the body in a functional design posture show the body aligned and balanced – see Table 14.2.

Maintaining a natural body alignment requires coordination of all the aforementioned parts of the body.

CREATE AND MAINTAIN A STABLE BASE

The position of the feet is the secret to safe handling. The handler's feet should be comfortably apart with one foot slightly in front of the other; this gives a wider base of support and stability in all directions. The position of the feet may also enable the handler to manage a surprise or unpredictable movement by the patient. Relaxing knees and hips with an offset base can improve balance. The offset feet position also creates a greater surface area as feet are kept in contact with the floor when knees

Table 14.2

Back	Shoulder, hip, knee and ankle joints vertically aligned with the line of gravity
	The pelvis in neutral alignment to support the 'S' curve of the spine and ready to move the body
Front	Head erect with straight chin level
	Efficiently weight bearing in a perfect balance
	Weight evenly balanced from front to back in the feet

Source: Wanless and Wanless, 2011

and hips are relaxed. Safe handling should always be within the handler's personal base, handling outside the base causes the handler to become unstable.

In order to demonstrate this exercise to outline the benefits of a stable base, ask three participants to stand and adopt one of the following stances:

- Feet side by side only slightly apart
- Feet side by side only with a wider base
- Feet slightly apart with one foot slightly in front of the other.

Another member of the group goes behind each of them and pushes them gently forwards in the lumbar area. The first two will not be able to hold their balance while the third will be able to absorb the movement by transferring weight forward and bending the forward knee.

BEND THE KNEES AND THE HIPS

When picking an object up from the floor a young child will bend their knees and hips, thereby allowing the quadriceps muscles to aid the movement – a natural movement we are all born with. Never handle in front of the knees as this makes the handler carry out the handling task at arm's length, and never handle to one side of the knees as this causes the spine to rotate when handling.

KEEP THE BACK NATURALLY STRAIGHT

Keeping the spine naturally straight allows it to act like a spring and absorb the body weight thereby assisting the main shock absorbers, and the smaller spinal muscles, to work to their full potential. Keeping a neutral position with the natural curves allows the spine to be a stable structure, by keeping parts of the spine either side of the line of gravity. However, a poker straight back allows the spine to become unstable as the small spinal muscles are unable to work to their potential. The spine should be kept naturally upright whenever it is possible, leaning forward, even a small degree, can add a considerable load onto the vertebral column. A naturally straight back allows significantly less stress on the spinal structures of the discs, facet joints and ligaments.

NEVER ROTATE OR TWIST THE SPINE

Twisting or a rotational movement of the spine reduces the effectiveness of the joints and muscles, decreasing the body's capacity to do work and thereby increasing the chance of an injury occurring. If the spine is bent forward and rotated there is a high level of compression on the spinal structures. If the spine has to be rotated, then the handler needs to reposition their feet as it is this that can cause the pelvis and shoulders not to be level. If the handler has to turn with the patient or twist the spine, then the handler should either pivot on their feet or reposition their feet, thereby reducing the rotational stress on the inter-vertebral discs.

Demonstrate this by asking participants to stand with their arms out straight and holding their hands together. Keeping their feet firmly placed on the floor ask them to rotate their torso without letting go of their hands, then check the amount of twist there is and the discomfort they feel. Ask them to repeat the movement only this time, as they move their torso, to either pivot on the heel of one foot and the balls of the other foot or move their feet to the side they are twisting to. Discuss which movement caused least discomfort. The answer will confirm that there is less discomfort when pivoting compared to keeping the feet static while twisting.

KEEP THE PERSON CLOSE TO YOUR TRUNK FOR AS LONG AS POSSIBLE

The distance of the person from the spine at waist height can be an important factor in the overall load on spine and back muscles. When moving and handling a system of levers comes into action, with the L5/S1spinal joint being the lower back lever joint. If a 20-pound load is lifted 20 inches from this lever point the compression on the spine, due to the horizontal distance, is 400lbs of compressive force. At the same time, your individual capability also decreases to approximately 50 per cent. If the object is moved further forward, causing the handler to lean forward at the waist, the handler's capability decreases. This pressure does not allow the spine to absorb the forces by compression but pulls the spinal joints apart and stretches the ligaments to their limit. It is essential to reduce the effect of excessive leverage; this is best achieved by taking up a position as close as possible to the patient. Always ensure a good firm grip on the patient as this may allay any fears they may have and increase their confidence in the handler's ability to assist them safely.

To demonstrate this, ask a participant to stand and hold in their hands a bag of sugar to the chest, extend the arms and ask if the weight feels as if it has increased. Keeping the arms out straight, give the instruction to lean slightly forward at the waist and again ask whether the weight feels as if it has increased. This movement should only be performed for a short time. The answer to your questions will be that the object feels as if it has increased in weight, proving the need to keep the patient or object as close to the handler as possible at all times throughout the movement.

ON COMMENCEMENT OF THE TASK

Raise the head and shoulders. This enables the carer to see any hazards they may have to step over or move around; at the same time it brings the cervical area of the spine into the correct position and ensures a naturally straight spine from the Coccyx up to Cervical 1.

At the same time, slight tension of the diaphragm, abdominal and pelvic floor muscles should be undertaken, which allows the abdominal pressure to remain constant. By so doing pressure is taken off the lumbar inter-vertebral discs.

LIFT AND LOWER WITH THE LEGS SMOOTHLY

Flexion at hips and knees allows the muscles in the legs to perform their task; quadriceps contract, hamstrings and calf muscles relax to allow the movement to take place. This helps to prevent stress on smaller spinal muscles. The movements should be controlled and smooth. Weight lifters use their leg muscles to lift by taking up the power position, allowing the muscles to work to their full potential.

USE YOUR BODY WEIGHT

Assisting a patient to stand or transfer requires not only muscle power but also the added assistance of the handler transferring their body weight. The basic principle behind using the handler's and the patient's body weight to transfer patients is to allow the use of momentum – otherwise known as Kinetic energy – to assist a handler to transfer a patient with minimal effort. The handler's hands and arms are used to guide a patient but the transferring of body weight and the muscle power is of major importance.

In order to demonstrate this, ask two participants to stand facing each other with one putting their hands on the other participant's shoulders. The person with their hands on the shoulders stands with their feet slightly apart and attempts to push the other person using their arms alone; meanwhile the person being pushed attempts to resist the movement. Then instruct the participant who is pushing to place their feet slightly apart, with one foot in front of the other. They should then attempt again to push the other person, only this time using their arms and their body weight by transferring from the back to the front foot. The movement of the participant who is pushing will overcome the resistance of the participant who is stationary, causing the stationary person to move.

The team must commence the movement on a predetermined signal – Ready, Steady, Stand/Sit/Slide – or whatever movement is required.

POINTS TO NOTE

The facilitator needs to have an awareness of the principles related to moving and handling and be up to date with the advancements in moving and handling practice. The facilitator is there to inform the student when they are compromising their health and wellbeing by not conforming to the physiological principles related to posture.

The basis of efficient patient handling is formed from the principles discussed above; the more the individual principles are used in a patient handling movement, the more efficient and risk free the movement will be.

CONCLUSION

Over the years there have been many changes in patient handling equipment – electric profiling beds and not fixed height beds are more common, hoists are available to lift patients rather than handlers, slide sheets are available in place of bed sheets – but the constant themes that have never changed in all those years are the basic principles of moving and handling. By following the basic patient handling principles, the handler is made aware of the dangers involved and is encouraged to adopt the safest position for handling. This does not mean that injuries due to moving and handling will cease to happen simply by following the rules.

Healthcare professionals work with the most unpredictable load in the world – a human being – and that is why they have the highest incidence rate of moving and handling injuries. However, by following the basic principles, handlers are putting themselves into the safest handling position they can adopt. Patient handling procedures have changed dramatically since the introduction of MHOR in 1992 (HSC, 2004), from full body lifting to using body weight, equipment and transfer. Perhaps over time procedures will change again, with the invention of more state-of-the-art equipment and innovations in moving and handling training; however, the principles of moving and handling will always continue to be the most important part of the movement of any patient or inanimate load.

SIMULATION SCENARIO

Assisted Sit to Stand

The patient will be assisted from the sitting position to standing, with the assistance of two handlers, from the side of a chair using a handling belt.
Points the facilitator should be looking for:

- Explanation of the procedure to the patient and their colleague
- That they first ascertain whether the patient can fully weight bear, by asking the patient if they can stand, then getting them to move themselves to the front of their chair and position their feet correctly
- The handling belt should be placed around the patient's waist and made comfortable and secure
- The handlers stand at the sides of the patient, as close as is possible
- The patient is encouraged either to place their hands on the arm of the chair or on the front of their thighs
- Each handler's rear foot should be in line with the patient's hip joint and their front foot slightly forward; both feet should face slightly into the patient, thus alleviating rotational stress

- The handlers hold on to the opposite rear handle on the belt with their inner arm, the outer arm is to hold on to the side handle of the belt
- The handler's body weight is on the slightly bent back foot and as they say ready, steady, stand to the patient, they transfer their body weight from the rear foot to the front foot and extend their legs
- On commencement of the task we should look for both handlers to raise their heads
- At the end of the movement the handlers should be in line with the patient, in the patient's peripheral vision.

REFERENCES

Department of Health (2002) *Campaign Launched to Cut Lost Days Through Back Injury.* London: Hutton.

Edlich, R.F., Winters, K.L., Hudson, M.A., Britt, L.D. and Long, W.B. (2004) 'Prevention of disabling back injuries in nurses by the use of mechanical patient lift systems', *Journal of Long-Term Effects of Medical Implants*, 14 (6): 521–3.

Health and Safety Commission (2004) *Manual Handling Operations Regulations 1992* (as amended). Sudbury: HSE Books.

Health and Safety Executive (1974) *Health and Safety at Work, etc Act.* London: HSE.

Health and Safety Executive (1998) *Provision and Use of Work Equipment Regulations.* London: HSE.

Health and Safety Executive (1998) *Lifting Operations and Lifting Equipment Regulations.* London: HSE.

Health and Safety Executive (2003) *Research Report 097. The Principles of Good Manual Handling: Achieving a Consensus.* Prepared by the Institute of Occupational Medicine for the Health and Safety Executive. London: HSE.

Leggett, P. (1998) *The Biomechanics of Human Movement – The Guide to the Handling of Patients,* revd 4th edn. Middlesex: National Back Pain Association.

Menzel, N., Brooks, S.M., Bernard, T.E. and Nelson, A. (2004) 'The physical workload of nursing personnel: association with musculoskeletal discomfort', *International Journal of Nursing Studies*, 41 (8): 859–67.

National Audit Office (2003) *A Safer Place to Work – Improving the Management of Health and Safety Risks to Staff in the NHS Trusts.* London: NAO.

Smedley, J., Inskip, H.,Trevelyan, F., Buckle, P., Cooper, C. and Coggon, D. (2003) 'Risk factors for incident neck and shoulder pain in hospital nurses', *Occupational and Environmental Management,* 66 (11): 864.

Wanless, S. and Wanless, G.S. (2011) 'Improving training and education in patient handling', *Nursing Times*, 107 (23): 17–19.

Workcover, NSW (1998) *Manual Handling Competencies for Nurses.* NSW, Australia: NSW Nurses' Association.

15

MANAGING CONFLICT IN HEALTHCARE

Stephen Wanless

Aim

The aim of this chapter is to give healthcare professionals an insight into, and strategies for dealing with, conflict within a healthcare setting.

Objectives

To give healthcare professionals the ability to:

- Develop an understanding of relevant responsibilities and develop practical risk recognition and reduction strategies when dealing with conflict through simulation
- Understand the relevance and necessity of reporting conflict
- Support personal and organisational learning
- Understand different ways to manage and de-escalate conflict.

INTRODUCTION

In today's healthcare environment, the potential for conflict among healthcare professionals exists as changes are occurring at a supersonic pace. The outcomes of conflict may affect patient care and are directly related to the effectiveness of the resolution. Clinical educators and staff development educators are essential in teaching resolution strategies that are currently being used in managing conflict and then to offer more effective resolution strategies.

Conflict in the healthcare arena has been defined as a dispute, disagreement, or difference of opinion related to the management of a patient involving more than one individual and requiring some decision or action (Studdert et al., 2003).

An estimated 20 per cent of time is spent dealing with conflict in the clinical setting (Aschenbrenner and Siders, 1999). Research indicates that healthcare professionals tend to take a passive approach to managing conflict, and that this approach is not in the best interests of contemporary work settings and the delivery of patient care (Tomey Marriner and Poletti, 1991; Tomey Marriner, 1995; Valentine, 1995). Managing conflict is equal to if not slightly higher in importance than planning, communication, motivation, and decision making (McElhaney, 1996).

During the current period of dynamic changes in healthcare systems, when healthcare professionals are forced to assume new roles, knowledge of conflict management strategies is particularly crucial.

Managing conflict in the workplace is a time-consuming but necessary task for the healthcare professional. Conflicts may exist between staff, and/or the healthcare team and the patient or patient's family. These conflicts may range from disagreements to major controversies that may lead to litigation or violence.

Conflicts have an adverse effect within the healthcare arena on productivity, morale and patient care. They may result in high employee turnover and certainly limit staff contributions and impede efficiency. Societies have significantly decreased their tolerance of disruptive behaviour. A group or organisation can now hold vicarious liability for condoning a hostile work environment if it fails to act when a complaint is made.

An essential element of teaching healthcare professionals how to manage conflict is the recognition that there are stages of conflict, with appropriate interventions at different stages. The stages of conflict can range from robust argument within a single meeting to longstanding opposing, entrenched positions of staff, administration, and the governing body.

Depending upon the culture or needs of the organisation and the type of conflict, an individual can practise and can use various communication skills and negotiation techniques to manage a conflict scenario. Healthcare professionals also need to be aware that a more formal process conducted by an experienced, skilled mediator may be more appropriate in managing complex conflicts.

Therefore, any conflict management simulation must allow for a variety of interventions – from informal methods such as persuasion, facilitation, conciliation or negotiation, to formal methods such as structured negotiation or mediations.

An effective conflict management simulation must be staged and proportional to allow for application consistent with the nature and seriousness of the conflict. It goes without saying that early recognition of conflict and an appropriate level of intervention must be a primary objective in managing any form of conflict.

Healthcare programmes focus mainly on developing critical skills and abilities when dealing with conflict. Bodine and Crawford (1998) state that training in managing conflict provides a basic understanding of the nature of conflict, an appreciation of how power and influence operate in all conflict situations, and an awareness of the role of culture in how we see and respond to conflict.

Not many pre-registration healthcare programmes include recognition of the ways people manage or respond to conflict, and the advantages and disadvantages of these ways. An extremely important programme component should involve providing students with social and emotional skills to prevent conflict and to reinforce their use of strategies to diffuse conflict in the clinical arena. Healthcare professionals also require training in the development of facilitation skills to maximise time efficiency and improve operations and compliance when dealing with conflict.

BACKGROUND TO THE SKILLS

By providing education and professional development to pre-registration healthcare professionals, and strategies for conflict management and dispute resolution, the academic can create synergy by merging solid conflict resolution processes with an environment rife with complex problems and motivated problem solvers. By creating shared meaning between universities and healthcare through simulation, we can begin to integrate interest-based processes into their existing activities.

With increasing expectations from the general public on the degree and standard of service they should expect to receive from the health service, coupled with the pressures from the government to supply those standards while cutting costs, healthcare professionals are experiencing conflict from every angle. Through the development of management of conflict skills in future clinicians, through appropriate role-play and simulation, healthcare organisations can begin to raise the level of dialogue from that of survival-of-the-fittest to that of collaboration and synergy.

The structure of training and education for healthcare professionals in managing conflict can take various forms. Creating education courses with this in mind can provide an educational forum and create an opportunity for intense learning outside of the clinical environment. Continuing education can take place at conferences and in workshops. Additionally, education can take place within the clinical setting through meetings, leadership development courses, and internal newsletters.

From within the healthcare organisation, education in conflict management can occur through integration of facilitation and mediation techniques into patient safety processes such as root cause analysis, process reviews, failure modes and effects analysis, disclosure conversations with patients, and team care conferences. Finding multiple ways to integrate skill development and process understanding into currently existing healthcare curricula is essential to the successful development of the field of healthcare conflict resolution.

To provide a framework for teaching conflict resolution to healthcare professionals, it helps to tie the principles of resolution to their clinical experience. Simple analogies during a facilitated session can help them see how something they are doing to resolve the conflict is similar to something they do clinically.

Healthcare professionals are excellent problem solvers. They are expert at analysing a problem, developing a strategy, locating resources and implementing the plan. This is how they are trained to care for patients. Using the analogy to patient care enables healthcare staff to grasp quickly the concepts associated with conflict management. The skills used to take care of patients can be honed to resolve conflicts and negotiate effectively.

A useful strategy for integrating skill development into a training session is to identify the steps in caring for a patient. The first step is assessment, then diagnosis of the disease or illness. Step three is creation of a treatment plan, followed by evaluation of the treatment and modification of the plan if necessary.

Given a clinical scenario, healthcare providers easily identify these steps in the process. They have difficulty applying the same process to conflict situations. If given a conflict scenario, for example, a dispute regarding visiting hours on the ward, most of the healthcare professionals will jump straight to diagnosis or treatment. They will describe the problem as, 'inconsistency in the enforcement of visiting hours' and therefore there must be a stricter policy and re-education about the policy. Assessment of what is leading to the inconsistent practice is not done. Analysing the situation and likening it to one of treating a patient without taking vital signs, listening to their lungs or looking at their lab work, helps clinicians grasp the importance of assessing the interests and needs at stake in a conflict situation.

In many cases, conflict in the workplace just seems to be a fact of life. We have all seen situations where different people with different goals and needs have come into conflict; and we've all seen the, often intense, personal animosity that can result.

The fact that conflict exists, however, is not necessarily a bad thing. As long as it is resolved effectively, it can lead to the personal and professional growth of an individual. Effective conflict resolution skills can make the difference between positive and negative outcomes.

The good news is that by assisting and educating healthcare professionals to resolve conflict successfully, you can solve many of the problems that it brought to the surface, as well as getting benefits that you might not at first expect:

- Increased understanding – The discussion needed to resolve conflict expands an individual's awareness of the situation, giving them an insight into how they can achieve their own goals without undermining those of other people
- Increased group cohesion – When conflict is resolved effectively, team members can develop stronger mutual respect and a renewed faith in their ability to work together
- Improved self-knowledge – Conflict pushes individuals to examine their goals in close detail, helping them understand the things that are most important to them, sharpening their focus, and enhancing their effectiveness.

If conflict is not handled effectively, the results can be damaging. Conflicting goals can quickly turn into personal dislike. Teamwork breaks down. Talent is wasted as people disengage from their work, and it's easy to end up in a vicious downward spiral of negativity and recrimination.

GOOD PRACTICE AND CURRENT UNDERSTANDING/THEORY

Despite an abundance of years in university, most healthcare professionals are lacking in basic skills necessary for resolving conflicts. Some of the skills that must be developed for effective conflict management in the clinical setting include: being present in the moment, listening for understanding, mutuality, openness, and reflection. Due to the chaos and complexity that exists in most healthcare environments, a majority of healthcare professionals are busy thinking about the next patient, how to get the next resource, when to fit in a test or procedure, when to eat or sleep, and responding to multiple distractions and interruptions. It is difficult truly to be present in the environment and listen to what others are saying at a deeper level.

Listening is typically restricted to information needed to move through the day and is rarely done at a level that enables understanding of a situation where there may be collaboration barriers resulting from fear, need for control, fatigue, a need to be right, or shame. Creating the ability to listen at a deeper level within a chaotic clinical environment is an essential skill for developing conflict resolution abilities in healthcare students.

Despite the descriptor 'healthcare team', there are relatively few times throughout the day when members of the interdisciplinary team function as a team. Most often, they are working as individual advocates for the patient through their role and only in rare instances, such as clinical emergencies, do they step out of that role and actually work together as a synergistic team. Turf battles, differences of knowledge level and experience, and rare opportunities for group conversation lead to a competitive atmosphere where everyone is struggling to do the right thing.

Development of the conflict resolution skill is essential for managing disputes and for preventing the shame/blame game that so frequently arises in the clinical setting. Fear of doing harm to the patient creates a great need for control of the patient and the environment, and can cause harm to the development of true teams. Demonstrating ways for developing through exercises and role playing is a great method for advancing the development of skilled clinicians.

Openness to alternative solutions is crucial to resolving complex problems. Developing this skill in healthcare students enables them to consider creative alternatives to a conflict situation. It is what enables them to think beyond 'a policy', 'a guideline', or 're-education' as the solution to their current conflict. Openness is necessitated by a trusting and supportive environment.

In a competitive environment where mistakes can be lethal, it is difficult for healthcare professionals to be open to the fact that their idea or answer could be wrong. There is a need to be right so as not to hurt the patient. This trait carries over into conflict situations where everyone has the right answer to the problem and has difficulty hearing conflicting solutions. On a broader level, with varied levels of training, there is a built-in tendency to believe that you know more than someone else because of specialty training, certification, and more experience or a higher position within the organisation. Developing openness across professions and across hierarchical levels is difficult but necessary to foster just agreements and lasting solutions.

Thomas and Kilmann (1977) identified five main styles of dealing with conflict that vary in their degrees of cooperativeness and assertiveness. They argued that people typically have a preferred conflict resolution style. However, they also noted that different styles were most useful in different situations. The Thomas-Kilmann Conflict Mode Instrument (TKI) helps you to identify which style you tend towards when conflict arises.

Thomas and Kilmann's five styles are: competitive, collaborative, compromising, accommodating, and avoiding (see Table 15.1).

Once you understand the different styles, you can use them to think about the most appropriate approach (or mixture of approaches) for the situation you are in. You can also think about your own instinctive approach, and learn how you need to change this if necessary. Ideally you can adopt an approach that meets the situation, resolves the problem, respects people's legitimate interests and mends damaged working relationships.

Lipsky and Avgar (2004) suggest that these procedures should be used when managing conflict as they are useful when attempting to solve 'individual' workplace conflict. This approach seeks to resolve workplace problems informally inside the organisation without having to use external mediators through a variety of mediation and/or arbitration procedures. Cutcher-Gershenfeld (2003) suggests that new practices need to be diffused within the organisation which can be used to address group-based problems and disputes in the healthcare setting.

Traditional collective bargaining processes are seen to be in need of reform so that they are less hostile and have a more 'interest-based' approach to conflict (Cutcher-Gershenfeld et al., 2007). Intensive information and consultation arrangements as well as approaches such as brainstorming and proactive communications around conflict are seen as necessary to encourage a more consensual atmosphere at the workplace, and to enable potential problems to be identified and addressed early (Rowe and Bendersky, 2003). This conflict resolution strategy respects individual differences while helping people avoid becoming too entrenched in a fixed position.

Collaboration and joint action are the by-words of interest-based negotiations (Barrett and O'Dowd, 2005). In educating healthcare professionals in resolving conflict it is important to ensure you highlight these rules:

- Make sure that good relationships are the first priority – As far as possible, make sure that you treat the other calmly and that you try to build mutual respect. Do your best to be courteous to one another and remain constructive under pressure
- Keep people and problems separate – Recognise that in many cases the other person is not just 'being difficult'; real and valid differences can lie behind conflictive positions. By separating the problem from the person, real issues can be debated without damaging working relationships
- Pay attention to the interests that are being presented – By listening carefully you will be much more likely to understand why the person is adopting their position

Table 15.1

Competitive	People who tend towards a competitive style take a firm stand, and know what they want. They usually operate from a position of power, drawn from things like position, rank, expertise, or persuasive ability. This style can be useful when there is an emergency and a decision needs to be made fast; when the decision is unpopular; or when defending against someone who is trying to exploit the situation selfishly. However, it can leave people feeling bruised, unsatisfied and resentful when used in less urgent situations.
Collaborative	People tending towards a collaborative style try to meet the needs of all people involved. These people can be highly assertive but, unlike the competitor, they cooperate effectively and acknowledge that everyone is important. This style is useful when you need to bring together a variety of viewpoints to get the best solution; when there have been previous conflicts in the group; or when the situation is too important for a simple trade-off.
Compromising	People who prefer a compromising style try to find a solution that will at least partially satisfy everyone. Everyone is expected to give up something and the compromiser also expects to relinquish something. Compromise is useful when the cost of conflict is higher than the cost of losing ground, when equal strength opponents are at a standstill, and when there is a deadline looming.
Accommodating	This style indicates a willingness to meet the needs of others at the expense of the person's own needs. The accommodator often knows when to give in to others, but can be persuaded to surrender a position even when it is not warranted. This person is not assertive but is highly cooperative. Accommodation is appropriate when the issues matter more to the other party, when peace is more valuable than winning, or when you want to be in a position to collect on this 'favour' you gave. However, people may not return favours and, overall, this approach is unlikely to give the best outcomes.
Avoiding	People tending towards this style seek to evade the conflict entirely. This style is typified by delegating controversial decisions, accepting default decisions, and not wanting to hurt anyone's feelings. It can be appropriate when victory is impossible, when the controversy is trivial, or when someone else is in a better position to solve the problem. However, in many situations this is a weak and ineffective approach to take.

- Listen first; talk second – To solve a problem effectively you have to understand where the other person is coming from before defending your own position
- Set out the 'Facts' – Agree and establish the objective, observable elements that will have an impact on the decision
- Explore options together – Be open to the idea that a third position may exist, and that you can get to this idea jointly.

By following these rules, you can often keep contentious discussions positive and constructive. This helps to prevent the antagonism and dislike which so often causes conflict to spin out of control.

POINTS TO NOTE

Conflict management exercises can be invaluable in clinical interactions, as they help you to determine the sources of conflict and give insights on how to build consensus and provide leadership through the conflict. Healthcare professionals and educators need to embrace conflict and use conflict management training to help to improve communication, deal with difficult people, build mediation skills, and create value and learning opportunities for students and employees.

We all experience conflict within our work. That is not surprising. Conflict is in all that we do, whether professionally or socially. Healthcare professionals need to recognise where the potential for conflict lies and what the likely responses to it should be.

As a result of the need to be right, there is a difficulty managing situations where it appears that the wrong choice was made or a system design flaw led to a bad outcome for the patient. Many conflicts in healthcare flare up around adverse outcomes or near misses with a patient's care. The quick jump to diagnosis usually results in a search for whom to blame for the bad outcome. The blame environment exacerbates the conflict by creating secrecy and shame. Individual reflection is a necessary skill for resolving these types of conflicts by enabling healthcare professionals to learn from the event and identify what they would do differently the next time. Organisationally, hospitals and healthcare organisations must also find a way to reflect on how to improve their processes rather than foster a punitive environment that adds fuel to conflicts or drives them underground until the next adverse event occurs.

Skill development in conflict management can enhance the role of the clinician in their current role and can assist managers in negotiating the complexity of their environments. In addition, skill training programmes can be designed specifically to develop healthcare professionals who are interested in becoming healthcare mediators or internal neutrals within healthcare organisations. Expanding the role of the mediator to include work within healthcare organisations will require the training of a core group of healthcare professionals who can integrate their clinical expertise with the practice of dispute resolution. Programmes with this purpose are relatively new and are developing momentum as more healthcare professionals become interested in the field of conflict resolution.

Clinical training does not prepare healthcare providers for working collaboratively. There is no training in facilitation, mediation, dialogue, or negotiation. There may be a few hours of training on group work or active listening, but that is geared toward a therapeutic outcome and rarely does the knowledge transfer to non-therapeutic situations. Core training in how to facilitate, how to intervene after a crisis, how to balance competing interests and how to manage culture change is imperative in integrating conflict resolution into the healthcare setting. Applying the processes of conflict resolution with clinical activities allows an immediate application of the principles of interest-based negotiation and mediation. It also enables clinicians to have a consistent method for doing non-clinical problem solving and for enhancing collaborative work relationships that carry back over into bedside care of the patient.

All training should be interactive and allow opportunity to apply the process to a clinical conflict. Healthcare professionals are 'doers' and learn well with applied exercises and the challenge of trying new skills. Applying the process to actual conflicts they are having in their workplace enables them to work through the conflict in a neutral setting and reinforces how to apply the process to their work environment. Processes that are beneficial in the clinical setting are facilitation, mediation, negotiation, appreciative inquiry, dialogue, and conciliation.

The object of utilising simulation in supporting this process is to allow students and healthcare professionals to learn to accept criticism, how to make their criticism constructive, and to see just how much complaining is hurled at people and that better solutions may be found through triggering discussion. A culture change is occurring in healthcare as the system grapples with ways to provide more care with fewer resources and improve safety through collaboration and better systems. For this change to be successful, healthcare organisations are going to need a critical mass of professionals with good conflict management skills and a means for integrating collaborative processes into their day-to-day operations. University programmes can fill that need by providing well-designed, interactive training programmes which enhance the ability of healthcare organisations to provide safe and effective care and which enable healthcare practitioners to regain hope that complex problems can have creative solutions.

CONCLUSION

Conflict in the workplace can be incredibly destructive to good teamwork. Managed in the wrong way, real and legitimate differences between people can quickly spiral out of control, resulting in situations where cooperation breaks down and the team's mission is threatened. This is particularly the case where the wrong approaches to assisting individuals in resolving conflict are used.

As an educator, when helping healthcare professionals to gain the skills in managing and calming these situations down, it helps to take a positive approach to teaching these skills, promoting courteous and non-confrontational discussion within the simulation setting, and maintaining the focus on issues provided by the simulation rather than on individual specific problems encountered when in practice. If this is done – as long as people listen carefully and explore facts, issues and possible solutions properly – the skill of managing conflict can be easily attained.

Allow the learner to think of a time when they responded positively in a situation of conflict and note what they did. What were they thinking or feeling at the time? What did they say? Was the conflict resolved so that all parties were committed to the solution? The thoughts and skills that they showed then may help them to deal with conflict next time.

By providing conflict awareness skills, team members can understand and anticipate possible conflict and where it might arise. The result is that when it does emerge, newly qualified healthcare professionals are not taken by surprise and have a range of lenses through which to perceive the problem. That, coupled with practical strategies for resolution, can help to cut the cost of conflict.

Conflict is an inevitable part of healthcare practice and arises from differences in needs, values and interests. What is vital is how an individual responds to and manages it. Allowing an individual to develop skills through simulation can help to highlight underlying issues and enhance understanding.

In the past, there has been little integration of managing conflict education as components implemented in university healthcare curricula. To encourage healthcare educators to consider using more in their work, this chapter has introduced an overview of managing conflict and has presented an example of simulation as a potential model for training. In addition, it discusses the possible challenges that can be successfully faced with this shift in focus.

Complaint

This scenario is about dealing with an aggressive relative who is demanding to know why their father is still in hospital. This can be a reasonably short scenario so can be run several times in succession if waiting students remain out of the room.

Resources Required

Equipment

- Two chairs
- Set of patient notes
- Desk
- Phone.

SIMULATION SCENARIO

Setting

Ward office 19.00 hours, on 17 October. Students will have had handover of relevant patients on ward.

Roles

There are three participants: the facilitator, student 1 and student 2 whose roles are detailed in Table 15.2.

Table 15.2

1 An angry relative (Son/Daughter of Edward French)	Role to be taken by facilitator – Very agitated, wants to complain about care that his/her father is receiving. 'Nothing seems to be happening', would rather get their father home as all hospitals do is 'kill patients with MRSA'
	Should use the word 'complaint' and initially direct focus towards 'student nurse'. Initially become more aggressive with each answer, perhaps leaning over staff. De-escalate if staff actions are reasonable and calming
2 Newly qualified nurse	Role to be taken by student 1 – to be advised they are trained nurse completing notes at a desk and are mentoring a student nurse
3 Student nurse	Role to be taken by student 2 – to be advised they are a student nurse being mentored by the staff nurse

Situation

The newly qualified nurse is sitting in the office looking at some paperwork when a relative comes in and begins to rant and rave about the care his/her father is receiving. The facilitator should use the word 'complaint', and should stand over the nurse and try to be reasonably intimidating. This scenario will run dependent on the reaction of the newly qualified nurse and the subsequent judgements of the facilitator, that is, does the nurse escalate or de-escalate the situation.

Areas for Discussion

- How does the student react?
- How does the newly qualified nurse handle this situation – do they protect the student?
- How could it have been handled differently?
- What are the important issues when dealing with an angry/upset relative?
- What shouldn't you do in this situation?
- Can these types of situations be avoided?
- How should complaints be handled?
- Who can the nurse call for help?

REFERENCES

Aschenbrenner, C.A. and Siders, C.T. (1999) 'Conflict management: managing low-to-mid intensity conflict in the healthcare setting, II', *Physician Exec*, 25: 44–50.

Barrett, J.T. and O'Dowd, J. (2005) *Interest-Based Bargaining: A User's Guide*. Oxford: Trafford Publishing.

Bodine, R.J. and Crawford, D. (1998) *The Handbook of Conflict Resolution Education: A Guide to Building Quality Programs in Schools*. San Francisco, CA: Jossey Bass.

Cutcher-Gershenfeld, J. (2003) 'How process matters: a five-phase model for examining interest-based bargaining', in T. Kochan and D. Lipsky (eds), *Negotiations and Change: From Workplace to Society*. Ithaca, NY: Cornell University Press, pp. 141–60.

Cutcher-Gershenfeld, J., Kochan, T., Ferguson, J.P. and Barrett, B. (2007) 'Collective bargaining in the twenty-first century: a negotiations institution at risk', *Negotiation Journal*, July: 249–65.

Lipsky, D.B. and Avgar, A.C. (2004) 'Research on employment dispute resolution: toward a new paradigm', *Conflict Resolution Quarterly*, 22 (1–2): 175–89.

McElhaney, R. (1996) 'Conflict management in nursing', *Nursing Management*, 27 (3): 49–50.

Rowe, M. and Bendersky, C. (2003) 'Workplace justice, zero tolerance and zero barriers', in T. Kochan and D. Lipsky (eds), *Negotiations and Change: From Workplace to Society*. Ithaca, NY: Cornell University Press, pp. 117–38.

Studdert, D.M., Burns, J.P., Mello, M.M., Puopolo, A.L., Truog, R.D. and Brennan, T.A. (2003) 'Nature of conflict in the care of pediatric intensive care patients with prolonged stay', *Pediatrics*, 112: 553–8.

Thomas, K. and Kilmann, R. (1977) 'Developing a forced-choice measure of conflict-handling behavior: the mode instrument', *Educational and Psychological Measurement*, 37 (2): 309–25.

Tomey Marriner, A. (1995) 'Strategies for managing conflict', *Journal of Multicultural Nursing & Health*, 2 (1): 6–9.

Tomey Marriner, A. and Poletti, P. (1991) 'Strategies for managing conflict', *International Nursing Review*, 38 (4): 118–20.

Valentine, P. (1995) 'Management of conflict: do nurses/women handle it differently?' *Journal of Advanced Nursing*, 22: 142–9.

16

DRUG ADMINISTRATION ERRORS

Robert Mapp

Aim

The aim of this chapter is to address four main areas:

- The most common types of errors
- Why errors occur (the influencing factors)
- Strategies to reduce errors
- Good practice for avoiding medication errors.

Objectives

By the conclusion of this chapter, the learner should be able to:

- Define what a medication error is and discuss definitions commonly used
- Discuss the most common types of errors
- Recognise why errors occur (influencing factors) and the strategies to reduce errors.

INTRODUCTION

The term 'medication error' can be defined as a mistake that happens in the stages of either prescribing, dispensing or administration of medication where a patient is injured, killed or potential harm could arise (Wolf, 1989).

Another definition of a medication error is any preventable event that may cause or lead to inappropriate medication use or patient harm while the medication is under the control of the health professional or patient (Jevon et al., 2010).

This chapter is aimed at all healthcare professionals who are involved in the administration of drugs to patients. The Department of Health (2005) states that any trained member of staff from health or social care can administer a medicine that has been prescribed by someone who is authorised to do so.

Many different healthcare professionals are legally permitted to prescribe and dispense medicines, and usually it is nurses who administer the drug to a patient. This indicates that it is the nurse who often bears the main responsibility for avoiding potential medication errors (Elliott and Liu, 2010).

BACKGROUND TO THE SUBJECT

Healthcare professionals are often involved in procedures and skills that affect patients, but the administration of medicines is a procedure that will be carried out on a day-to-day basis. Some drug rounds could take up to two hours to complete and will be performed at least three times a day. This opens up the risk for potential errors to be made on an almost regular basis (Elliott and Liu, 2010).

The administration of medicines is seen as a crucial role for healthcare professionals within the healthcare sector. For inpatients, medicines are normally prescribed, dispensed and administered by doctors, pharmacists and nurses. These can range from giving simple oral medication such as paracetamol tablets, to more complex mixtures of medicines to be given intravenously (Tiziani, 2002).

The focus of this chapter is medication errors and these can be looked at in several ways. They are no longer seen as a simple error where the wrong drug has been given to a patient. Medication errors can occur from the initial prescribing and dispensing of the drug, to the administration process falling down on account of several possible factors.

Medication errors are one of the main causes of morbidity and mortality of patients who are hospitalised (Elliott and Liu, 2010). This shows clearly that it is imperative to try and reduce medication errors, so that patients receive safe and efficient care around the medication administered (Brady et al., 2009; Agyemang and While, 2010).

As well as a professional duty of care, there is also a legal aspect. Where a healthcare professional's actions or omissions could cause harm to another person, this can be classed as negligence (Dimond, 2004).

THE MOST COMMON TYPES OF ERRORS

Medication errors can occur at any stage of a process; this includes areas such as prescribing, dispensing, distribution and administration. All of these areas need adequate communication between healthcare professionals and with patients (Department of Health (DH), 2004).

Another area where errors commonly occur is the omission of drugs – failing to give a drug for whatever reason – or not monitoring adverse reaction in a patient. Agyemang and While (2010) state that an omission error is where a healthcare professional fails to administer the prescribed dose without good reason.

Drugs errors can be caused by any stage of the above process breaking down. There are three stages at which errors can more commonly occur: prescribing, dispensing and administrating.

Prescribing medication is predominantly the role of a doctor, although other healthcare professionals may do this through their extended role. Errors can occur at this stage, with the writing of an incorrect prescription. This could be due to a practitioner prescribing the wrong drug or, more commonly, not indicating the correct dose required on the prescription chart. Issues can also arise from the illegibility of handwriting on the actual prescription or drug chart.

Dispensing medication is predominantly the role of a pharmacist; individual pharmacists are responsible for dispensing drugs to patients going home or to departments or wards. Errors can occur if this procedure is not carried out correctly. For example, the drug dosage may not be dispensed correctly or bottles or drug boxes may be wrongly labelled. Contributing factors of a drug error involving dispensing include late deliveries and lack of 24-hour cover of pharmacists to wards (Brady et al., 2009).

Administration is carried out the majority of the time by qualified nurses. As nurses are often the last point in this process, it is frequently nurses who administer drugs to patients (Department of Health (DH), 2004). This is the point where the majority of errors can occur. This is because it is the last step before the patient actually takes the drug, and because it is carried out so frequently on a daily basis by nearly all nurses (Gladstone, 2008). There are different types of errors that can occur, by administering:

- the wrong drug
- at the wrong time
- by the wrong route
- in the wrong dose
- to the wrong patient.

The administration of medicines includes taking the prescription with the drugs trolley to the patient's bedside and traditionally carrying out the five rights (Five Rs) of medication administration: the Right patient, Right route, Right dose, Right medicines and Right time (Elliott and Liu, 2010; Crouch and Chapelhow, 2008).

We can break this process down further. The right patient is ensured by checking that the patient's hospital wrist band coincides with the prescription chart. Both the prescription chart and the patient's wrist band should include their name, date of birth and an individual National Health Service (NHS) number which is specific to the individual patient.

The correct route of administration is ensured by checking the route indicated on the prescription chart and the correct clinical knowledge of the healthcare practitioner. If unsure, the British National Formulary (BNF) should always be checked. The BNF is essential reading for healthcare professionals in regard to medication management (Pountney, 2010).

The right dose is again checked against the prescription chart and correlated with the BNF, if unsure. The healthcare professional administering the drug needs to ensure that the dose taken out of the packet or in the syringe is correct. For example, if 1 gram of paracetamol is prescribed, then the healthcare professional needs to ensure that 2 × 500 milligram tablets have been dispensed.

The correct medicine is ensured by again checking that the prescription correlates with the actual drug dispensed. The healthcare professional also needs to ensure that the patient is not allergic to the medication and that it is indeed the correct medicine for the purpose for which it is intended. Finally, the right time looks at the intended time that the drug should be administered to the patient – ensuring it is within the administration time frame.

WHY DO ERRORS OCCUR (INFLUENCING FACTORS)

Why do medication errors occur? This is a vital question as the main course of action to reduce any risk is to focus on and identify what causes the errors in the first place. While the vast majority of medication prescribed and administered is done so safely, the risk involved is always present and – unavoidably – some mistakes and errors will happen (Department of Health (DH), 2004).

Medication errors are common but still often go unreported; in the United Kingdom as many as 10 per cent of inpatients may experience a drug error (Elliott and Liu, 2010). There are two types of medication errors classed as adverse events and near misses; near misses are salutary lessons as no actual harm has come to a patient due to these mistakes.

All procedures and skills carry an element of risk, but it could be argued that medication administration on the whole carries the most risk, as it is undertaken numerous times a day by almost all nurses (Elliott and Liu, 2010). One of the main reasons for medication errors is that healthcare professionals are human and, by default, errors will occur (Elliott and Liu, 2010). Many errors are put down to human slip ups, mistakes or just lapses in concentration, while others are attributed to system failures. Once an error has occurred the main aim must be to ensure that the error is reported so that an attempt can be made to pinpoint and understand the cause of the error (Naylor, 2002). Slips or lapses in concentration can be classed as different to an actual mistake, but are no less excusable and could result in the same outcome – death or injury to a patient (Naylor, 2002).

Lack of knowledge of a particular drug can lead to an error occurring through the delivery of the wrong dose, or via the wrong route and even administering the wrong drug to the patient. As Wiseman and Volans (2007) point out, potential interactions between two or more drugs are very common. Medication errors have also occurred when the particular drug given has not been recorded or signed for by the registered practitioner, or doses have either been given twice by mistake or omitted for the wrong reasons (Department of Health (DH), 2005).

Medication errors occur in several potential problem areas; individual errors in prescribing, dispensing and, particularly, administrating will all result in medication errors. If national and local policy and procedures are not followed, this will ultimately lead to mistakes. Other individual areas include lack of clinical knowledge and lapses in concentration.

Systemic failures are those areas individuals cannot control, such as staffing issues and workload, which could all ultimately lead to errors occurring. A lot of incidents are multifaceted and are due to system failures within the NHS or local policies that are not being followed. Some common causes are failure to identify the patient correctly, dose calculation errors, workload issues and poor clinical knowledge (Department of Health (DH), 2004).

STRATEGIES TO REDUCE ERRORS – GOOD PRACTICE

In 2001 the government set up the National Patient Safety Agency (NPSA). This was to ensure that there was a single body responsible for reporting and learning systems with regard to adverse incidents in the NHS. Medication errors are obviously a part of NPSA's clear remit to improve patient safety (Department of Health (DH), 2004; Crouch and Chapelhow, 2008).

Medication errors will occur when either human or system factors affect the prescribing or administration of medicines to patients. This produces an unintended and potentially fatal or harmful outcome. The Department of Health produced a report in 2004 (DH, 2004) called *Building a Safer NHS for Patients* which looked at the risk factors in all stages of the medication process.

Medication administration is dependent on a number of factors to ensure accuracy, and those individuals carrying out this procedure need to be trained to do so accurately. Risk management must also be built into the process of drug administration. Other areas for consideration are clear procedures for drug administration, the double checking of drugs where appropriate, safe storage of all medicines and, finally, the use of technology to support the process (Department of Health (DH), 2004).

The *Building a Safer NHS for Patients* report (DH, 2004) concluded that the main aim is to find the common causes of medication issues and decide how these can be prevented. Some of these issues include ensuring that all patients with allergies have a red wrist band stating this, and that appropriate staff training must be in place. Individuals should be assessed as competent before they administer drugs independently. Medication administration should be covered by every new member of staff to the NHS on induction if they are to be involved in the process.

There are a number of issues that could and need to be tackled while looking at how to reduce medication errors within the NHS. The Department of Health

(DH, 2005) states that newly qualified doctors and nurses need to undertake a strenuous induction programme that covers prescribing and administrating medicines respectively. Supporting this statement is a further belief that healthcare professionals need to have a greater knowledge base with regard to medication, pharmacology and drug interactions in order to safely and effectively administer and prescribe medication.

Policy and procedures need to be in place, and followed, for medication errors to be reduced. For nurses, the five rights of medication administration (the Five Rs, as listed above) need to be followed strictly – performing the basic checking of a patient's wrist band against the prescription chart, along with communication between professionals and the patient, will go a long way to ensuring correct practice is adhered to (Department of Health (DH), 2004).

GOOD PRACTICE – HOW TO AVOID MEDICATION ERRORS

No healthcare professional intentionally sets out to harm a patient or make a medication error. The vast majority of medication prescribed or administered to patients is done so without incident and with all policies and procedures adhered to in a correct manner.

The following list highlights several areas of good practice which have been adopted by various NHS trusts and which further add to this process of error reduction:

- Five rights
- Tabard system – the administrator wearing a red tabard to ensure they are not disturbed when completing a drug round
- Medication administration records (MARs)
- Self medication – when a patient administers their own drugs as they would in their home setting.

All healthcare professionals involved in the medication process, from prescribing to administering, need to be aware and understand actions, contraindications and drug physiology. This needs to be looked at in relation to the patient's condition and knowledge of the diagnosis. The Department of Health (DH, 2004) argues that it is essential that undergraduate courses address medication issues, including pharmacology and drug interactions.

Ideally drug prescriptions should be computerised as this bypasses problematic issues such as illegible handwriting. Alerts will also flash up on the system to indicate allergies that have already been programmed in and to tell the practitioner if the drug has already been administered. This system has already proved very successful and started to reduce the amount of errors (Naylor, 2002).

Medication Administration Records (MARs) are currently used in most NHS Trusts in the UK. These are computerised prescription sheets where the details of drugs given and omitted are recorded by the healthcare practitioner (Department of Health (DH), 2004).

Other drug administration good practice tips – simple dos and don'ts – include:

- never give a drug that has been prepared by someone else
- never leave a drug trolley opened and unattended or unlocked
- do not leave drugs at the patient's bedside
- observe the patient taking the medication
- note allergy bracelets as they are extremely important and should clearly display the name of the drug that patient is allergic to
- even if the patient is not wearing a wrist band, you need to double check that they have no known allergies (Preston, 2004).

POINTS TO NOTE

When teaching this subject or discussing medication errors, some main areas to consider are:

- The correct policies and procedures for the administration, prescribing and dispensing of medicines
- Potential errors that could occur
- Why individuals cut corners
- Highlighting clinical and pharmacological knowledge.

CONCLUSION – IMPORTANT POINTS ABOUT THE SKILL

The vast majority of drug administration is provided and given to patients in the correct manner which is both safe and effective. The challenge is to build on this good practice and for NHS trusts to continue to make improvements in the systems that guide the way that healthcare professions prescribe, dispense and administer medicines to patients.

Medication errors do occur and it is impossible to eradicate mistakes completely. However, the focus should be on the reduction of errors to an absolute minimum. The main process is to identify good practice and carry through on its implementation, with the aim of reducing medication error.

Many of the reasons why medication errors occur have been discussed, with both individual errors and system failures playing a part. It is down to local NHS trusts to ensure that healthcare professionals follow the correct procedures and policies in place with regard to the dispensing, prescribing and administration of medicines.

There is a clear need for individuals to take greater ownership of their own practice, ensuring that their clinical and pharmacological knowledge is up to date, utilising resources like the British National Formulary (2011) and embracing the new systems set up to reduce errors, such as computerised prescribing systems.

Medication Error

This scenario asks the nurse to address a situation where medication has been left at the bedside of a patient and found by an HCA.

Equipment Required

- Medicine pot containing various tablets
- Administration chart relating to patient
- Desk
- Two chairs.

Setting

Nursing station: 09.30 hours; general medical ward.

Roles

There are three participants: the facilitator, student 1 and student 2 whose roles are detailed in Table 16.1.

Table 16.1

Healthcare Assistant (HCA)	Role to be taken by facilitator. The HCA will approach the two nurses and explain they have found some tablets for Mr Shielspeck on his bedside table. State that you are going to give them to him now but just want to let them know. You think you are being very helpful and are very insistent. If you are told you cannot administer the tablets you will ask why
	You have asked the patient and he doesn't think he has had any tablets today
Staff Nurse 1	Role to be taken by student. Will have to deal with the situation presented to you by the HCA. Second nurse is available for support
Staff Nurse 2	Role to be taken by student. Will have to deal with the situation presented to you by the HCA. First nurse is available for support

Situation

An HCA approaches the nurse's station and states that, while helping Mr Shielspeck have a wash at the bedside, they have found a pot of medicines on his bedside table. The HCA asks if they should get the patient to take them now. They have the administration chart with them that shows that the medication is signed for from 07.00 hours by a nurse who was on the night shift but who has now gone home. The two staff nurses must deal with the situation appropriately.

NB: Refer to the following NMC *Standards for Medicine Management* (Nursing and Midwifery Council, 2007).

Standard 8:

As a registrant, in exercising your professional accountability in the best interests of your patients:

- You must be **certain** of the identity of the patient to whom the medicine is to be administered.
- You must check that the patient is not allergic to the medicine before administering it.
- You must know the therapeutic uses of the medicine to be administered, its normal dosage, side effects, precautions and contraindications.
- You must be aware of the patient's plan of care (care plan/pathway).
- You must check that the prescription or the label on the medicine dispensed is clearly written and unambiguous.
- You must check the expiry date (where it exists) of the medicine to be administered.
- You must have considered the dosage, weight where appropriate, method of administration, route and timing.
- You must administer or withhold in the context of the patient's condition (e.g. digoxin not usually to be given if pulse below 60) and co-existing therapies (e.g. physiotherapy).
- You must contact the prescriber or another authorised prescriber without delay where contraindications to the prescribed medicine are discovered, where the patient develops a reaction to the medicine, or where assessment of the patient indicates that the medicine is no longer suitable (see Standard 25).
- You must make a clear, accurate and immediate record of all medicine administered, intentionally withheld, or refused by the patient, ensuring the signature is clear and legible; it is also your responsibility to ensure that a record is made when delegating the task of administering medicine.

In addition:

- Where medication is not given, the reason for not doing so must be recorded.
- You may administer with a single signature any Prescription Only Medicine (POM), general sales list (GSL) or Pharmacy (P) medication.

Standard 17 states that:

A registrant is responsible for the delegation of any aspects of the administration of medicinal products and they are accountable to ensure that the patient or carer/care assistant is competent to carry out the task.

Standard 19 states that:

In delegating the administration of medicinal products to unregistered practitioners, it is the registrant who **must** apply the principles of administration of medicinal products as listed above. They may then delegate an unregistered practitioner to assist the patient in the ingestion or application of the medicinal product.

Standard 24 states that:

As a registrant, if you make an error you must take any action to prevent any potential harm to the patient and report as soon as possible the prescriber, your line manager or employer (according to local policy) and document your actions. Midwives should also inform their named Supervisor of Midwives.

Areas for Discussion

- Do the nurses check the administration chart?
- Potentially the drugs had been signed for but not administered
- Can the nurses be sure the tablets are meant for this patient?
- Can the nurses be sure that these tablets were meant to be the 7 a.m. dose?
- NMC guidelines above state that if the medication is not given, the reasons why not should be documented
- Who was accountable for ensuring the medication was taken by the patient? (original administering nurse)
- Who is accountable for leaving the medication on the cabinet? (original administering nurse)
- What should happen to the tablets found? (discard)
- Can the nurse allow the HCA to give the medication? No – for all of the identified reasons above, however Standard 19 can be considered at other times
- What are the implications for the patient having or not having these tablets now?
- Did the nurses report this incident to the medical team or senior nurse? (Standard 24 and whistle blowing).

REFERENCES

Agyemang, R. and While, A. (2010) 'Medication errors: types, causes and impact on nursing practice', *British Journal of Nursing*, 19 (6): 380–5.

Brady, A., Malone, A. and Fleming, S. (2009) 'A literature review of the individual and system factors that contribute to medication errors in nursing practice', *Journal of Nursing Management*, 17: 679–97.

British National Formulary (Joint Formulary Committee) (2011) *62nd Edition*. London: British Medical Association and Royal Pharmaceutical Society.

Crouch, S. and Chapelhow, C. (2008) *Medicines Management: A Nursing Perspective*. Harlow: Pearson Education.

Department of Health (DH) (2004) *Building a Safer NHS for Patients: Improving Medication Safety*. London: DH. Available on: http://www.dh.gov.uk [accessed 12 December 2010].

Department of Health (DH) (2005) *Medicines Matters*. London: DH. Available on: http://www.dh.gov.uk/prod_consum_dh/groups/dh_digitalassets/@dh/@en/documents/digitalasset/dh_4106226.pdf [accessed 12 December 2010].

Dimond, B. (2004) 'Accountability and medical products 2: civil law', *British Journal of Nursing*, 13 (4): 217–19.

Gladstone, A. (2008) 'Drug administration errors: a study into the factors underlying the occurrence and reporting of drug errors in a district general hospital', *Journal of Advanced Nursing*, 22 (4): 626–37.

Elliott, M. and Liu, Y. (2010) 'The nine rights of medication administration: an overview', *British Journal of Nursing*, 19 (5): 300–5.

Jevon, P., Payne, E., Higgins, D. and Endacott, R. (eds) (2010) *Medicines Management*. Oxford: Wiley-Blackwell.

Naylor, R. (2002) *Medication Errors: Lessons for Education and Healthcare*. Oxford: Radcliffe Medical Press.

Nursing and Midwifery Council (2007) *Standards for Medicine Management*. London: NMC. Available on: http://www.nmc.org [accessed 12 December 2010].

Pountney, D. (2010) 'Effective administration of medicines', *Nursing and Residential Care*, 12 (4): 170–4.

Preston, R. (2004) 'Drug errors and patient safety: the need for a change in practice', *British Journal of Nursing*, 13 (2): 72–8.

Tiziani, A. (2002) *Harvards Nursing Guide to Drugs*, 6th edn. Marrickville: Mosby.

Wiseman, H. and Volans, G. (2007) *Drugs Handbook*. Basingstoke: Palgrave Macmillan.

Wolf, Z.R. (1989) 'Medication errors and nursing responsibility', *Holistic Nursing Practice*, 4 (1): 8–17.

17

INTERVIEW TECHNIQUES

Katie Holmes and Nathalie Turville

Aim

To understand the importance of interview techniques as an essential skill that contributes to a successful career.

Objectives:

- To define 'employability'
- To discuss the skills required for each stage of the interview process
- To identify strategies for delivering a mock application and interview process with healthcare students.

INTRODUCTION TO INTERVIEW TECHNIQUES

This chapter deals with the skill of being able to perform well at interviews. The importance of this skill becomes apparent when considered within the wider context of employability. 'Employability' is a term used in Higher Education. Students, Higher Education Institutions (HEIs), and employers are all keen that graduates have the skills to be able to enter and be successful in the job market. A widely adopted definition of employability is:

> a set of achievements – skills, understandings and personal attributes – that make graduates more likely to gain employment and be successful in their chosen occupations, which benefits themselves, the workforce, the community and the economy. (Yorke and Knight, 2006: 3)

BACKGROUND TO THE SKILL

Employability skills are about more than just being able successfully to land that first job following graduation. They are a range of skills that will be of value throughout the individual's career.

> According to a survey of five hundred Directors in Oct 2007, when recruiting, 64% said graduates' employability skills were more important to their organisation than the specific occupational, technical or academic knowledge/skills associated with the graduate's degree (Johnstone and Willis, 2010: 2)

While healthcare is a sector where more focus is on the specific occupational knowledge and technical skills of employees than other sectors, there is recognition of the increasing importance of employability skills in this field. Skills for Health (2011), the skills council for the sector, argues that employability skills should be highly sought after by health sector employers. This is because they are the key to developing a skilled and flexible workforce, made up of individuals who can, for example, solve problems, make effective decisions, communicate, prioritise their workload, and are willing continuously to learn and grow.

The skills employers are looking for fall into four main categories: self-reliance skills (such as self-awareness, using initiative, networking, willingness to learn and action planning), people skills (team-working, leadership, communication and interpersonal skills), general employment skills (problem-solving, flexibility, IT literacy and commitment) and specialist skills (occupationally specific skills/knowledge). The job interview provides the space where in-depth exploration of the candidate's employability skills takes place and for this reason it is crucial that students have the opportunity to develop and practice interview techniques.

EXAMPLES OF GOOD PRACTICE AND CURRENT UNDERSTANDING

HEIs recognise their responsibility to ensure there are opportunities for students to develop their employability skills, self-awareness and confidence to be able to promote their skills during job interviews. While healthcare courses such as nursing offer substantial opportunities for students to develop their employability skills through the balance of clinical placements and academic study, the importance of providing opportunity for students to develop interview techniques should not be overlooked. Students may pass all of the requirements of their course and be competent and efficient, but if they cannot articulate and demonstrate their skills effectively to employers they will not be successful in gaining employment.

Psychological studies have been carried out as to whether attendance at interview coaching sessions does in fact have an impact on students' subsequent performance at job interviews. Maurer et al. report in their findings that 'When individual differences were controlled, coaching attendance was positively related to ... the interview performance' (2001: 715). Research such as this reinforces the argument for incorporating interview techniques sessions within HE courses, or at the very least making them available as an option for students.

By the term 'interview techniques' we are referring to the process of preparing for the interview, the skills involved in performing well during the interview itself, and reflecting/evaluating once the interview is over. This further encompasses a range of skills – the ability to research both the employer and current issues in the job sector; to be able to reflect on one's strengths, knowledge and experience and match this to the employer's requirements; to be aware of body language, have the ability of articulation and clear expression; and finally the ability honestly to critique oneself. Underlying all of these are the important qualities of self-belief and self-confidence, without arrogance.

Research in social psychology around the initial perceptions and decisions made about individuals during the first moments of meeting reinforces the importance of making a good first impression during job interviews. In their study, Barrick et al. (2010) found that candidates making better initial impressions received more job offers and higher interview scores: '... information communicated through something as simple as a handshake, a smile or the manner of dress can influence impressions' (Barrick et al., 2010: 1163). Interestingly enough, the initial impressions formed by employers went further than just an instinctive liking for an individual; they also formed a favourable impression of the interviewee's competence. This impression was unlikely to alter during the course of the interview. Therefore, the first few seconds of the interview can determine its outcome – a key message to be reinforced to students.

There is a wide range of literature available with advice on preparing for interviews, some key messages being referred to repeatedly. Material from the Association of Graduate Careers Advisory Services (AGCAS), the Royal College of Nursing (RCN), and *Nursing Times* all refer to the following key factors in ensuring success at interviews. (Web addresses are available in the References section at the end of the chapter.)

PREPARATION

The preparation for interview starts with researching the job role and the organisation thoroughly. This is especially important if students have already worked for the NHS Trust before – or even in the same ward/clinic/department – as they may feel that their experience means they do not need to carry out any further research. Feedback from NHS recruiting staff suggests that often such candidates lack wider knowledge about the Trust, for example, new developments taking place, the mission statement and key staff. It is recommended that candidates take advantage of the offer of a pre-visit to help with this preparation. It allows candidates to ask questions that they may not wish to raise at interview – for example, frequency of night duty – and to explore the reality of working in that area from the perspective of a qualified practitioner. In addition, it gives the candidate the opportunity to create a positive first impression. However, this is a two-way process and it may be that following an informal visit and meeting staff, the prospective candidate may choose not to proceed with their application. Preparation is also about self-knowledge – being able to reflect on the skills developed through experiences in previous employment, through academic study, and outside interests and hobbies, and relating these skills to the requirements of the post for which they have applied.

PRACTICE

Spending time rehearsing answers is invaluable. The STAR technique (displayed in Box 17.1) is widely advocated in careers guidance circles as an effective structure for answers (Morton-Holmes, 2009).

BOX 17.1

Situation	Describe the **Situation**.
Task	What was your **Task**?
Action	What **Action** did you take
Result	What were the **Results**?

PRACTICALITIES

The importance of ensuring all the practicalities are dealt with, such as what to wear and gathering together any documentation needed, cannot be overstated. The outfit chosen by the candidate should project a professional image but also allow the candidate to feel comfortable. Planning the journey and allowing for parking is also essential; parking at NHS Trusts is notoriously difficult and being late for an interview as a result of not being able to find a parking space does not create a favourable impression. It is also helpful to have the contact details of the Trust available should an emergency arise. If public transport is being used, it is important to be familiar with the routes and times, allowing ample time for the journey.

BODY LANGUAGE

The candidate should be aware of their own body language and how confidence, positivity and professionalism can all be conveyed through non-verbal communication. Simarly, the ability to read the body language of the interviewer and pick up on any non-verbal cues is also valuable (Littleford et al., 2004). Considerable research has been undertaken around the impact of body language during interactions between human beings and, as with the point on initial first impressions, the importance of non-verbal messages should not be overlooked.

AWARENESS OF THE VARIOUS TYPES OF QUESTIONS WHICH CAN ARISE

Scenario-based questions and competency-based questions, and some of the most widely asked questions, should be researched. This will help with preparation and practice. The HEI careers department should be able to provide sample questions for the different health professions and some sample questions are available at the end of this chapter.

REFLECTION

The practice of reflection following a job interview is essential if the candidate is to learn from the experience. The candidate needs to evaluate their performance and identify what went well and the areas for improvement, analyse the interview process and plan for future interviews (Littleford et al., 2004).

POINTS TO NOTE

As well as the material from organisations mentioned above, such as AGCAS, the careers department of the HEI will have a range of their own materials. Indeed, many have developed specialist booklets and resources relating to interview techniques for health students based on good practice and feedback from local NHS Trusts. It is highly recommended that the careers department is involved when planning sessions on interview techniques. As well as providing material they are often able to facilitate delivery of the sessions. Close collaboration between the academic staff and the careers department is invaluable in obtaining a good balance – on the one hand the knowledge and experience of the health sector and, on the other, the expertise in career management.

The simulation included in this chapter involves a mock application process starting with an application form, and then a mock interview following the shortlisting of appropriate candidates. Educators can choose whether to follow this process or to focus solely on the mock interview itself. Whichever method is chosen it is useful to point out that completing this exercise in itself will help students to develop employability skills.

CONCLUSION

Increasingly, employers are looking for a range of skills, knowledge and attitudes in candidates and it is essential that HEIs provide students with the opportunity to develop these employability skills throughout their time on the course. These skills will need to be articulated in the application and interview process, therefore students must be prepared so that they are able to sell themselves and be successful at interview. There is a significant amount of general and profession-specific guidance on interview preparation available for academic staff and students; however, practising techniques familiarises students with the application and interview processes, enables them to gain confidence in selling themselves and allows for feedback and reflection on their performance. The use of the interview techniques simulation provides the opportunity for close collaboration between academic, clinical and careers staff. It also ensures that students are ready to enter the job market, equipped with skills that will be used throughout their career.

SIMULATION SCENARIO

Interview

Introduction

The simulation enables the student to experience the application and interview process from the completion of the application form, preparing for interview, the actual interview and then receiving feedback and self-evaluation of their performance at interview. This simulation is staged over a minimum of four weeks to enable the student to fully engage in the process.

Learning Outcomes

At the end of the simulation the students will be able to:

- Complete an application form effectively
- Prepare for an interview
- Demonstrate suitable knowledge, skills and attitudes at an interview
- Critically evaluate their performance following an interview.

Resources Required for the Simulation

Equipment

- A job advert, job description, person specification and application form. One way to obtain these documents is to download them relating to an appropriate post from www.jobs.nhs.uk and they may be used as a template for the exercise, with adaptations to suit local requirements. The NHS Jobs website is the leading on-line recruitment service in the UK for NHS posts for all healthcare professionals.
- List of questions. The questions can include introductory ice-breakers, questions relating to the organisation and post applied for, professional development, skills (personal and clinical) and any 'hot topics'. The use of scenarios is a popular way to assess knowledge and attitudes. Six to eight questions per 20-minute interview should be appropriate. Clinical staff may be able to identify 'hot topics' for questions. It is important that the questions also reflect the job description and person specification.
- Letter inviting student to interview (optional). The letter may be an adaptation of one sent by a Human Resources Department. In the letter, the interviewers' names and title or role are included, plus any instructions about anything to bring to interview (e.g. portfolio) and where to report if necessary. The facilitator may also request the student to acknowledge the invitation to interview and their confirmation of attendance. This familiarises students with the different stages of the application and interview process and enables the facilitator to identify if the student has followed instructions. An example is available at the end of the chapter.
- Sheet for scoring performance at interview. This may be devised by the teaching team or based on a template used in clinical practice. An example is available at the end of the chapter.
- Post-interview review sheet for students (optional). This can be devised by the teaching team. It should cover the main elements of an interview: preparation, presentation, answering and asking questions, concluding the interview. An example can be found in Littleford et al., 2004.

Roles

Facilitators to act as interviewers. These facilitators may be academic staff, however clinical staff involved in recruitment or HEI careers advisers are often willing to participate in the simulation. There should be two facilitators to act as interviewers for each interview. If clinical staff are participating in the simulation and the students are aware of their role and their employing Trust, then it can help the student in their preparatory research and in formulating their responses to questions.

The facilitators who are acting as interviewers will be providing constructive feedback on the application form and interview. In their role, they will need to ensure that they are dressed appropriately for conducting interviews and maintain a more formal manner throughout the interview. There may be a training need regarding current recruitment techniques and the HEI careers adviser may be invited to provide updates and training.

Students will be playing the role of interviewees.

Setting

A small office or classroom where the interview can be conducted is required and, if possible, there should be an area where the student can wait prior to their interview.

Discussion Points and Areas for Consideration to Assist Facilitator

The job description, person specification and application form will be given to each student who wishes to participate in the simulation. A deadline for submission will be provided and no applications after this date should be considered. This emphasises to students the importance of adhering to deadlines and completing forms in a timely fashion. Students need to be aware when submitting real applications that if Trusts have received a sufficient number of applications for shortlisting, they will close the job advert. The student will complete the application form as though it were for an actual job, students can be told to treat the fictitious job advert and Trust as the actual Trust at which they have had their placements or where they would wish to work. The supporting information must reflect the person specification and the post for which they are applying.

In support of this, teaching about completion of application forms and the interview process will need to be provided if it has not already been delivered earlier in the programme. The HEI careers adviser will be able to provide resources and possible teaching on these areas.

The students will be informed of the deadline for the application form. They need to be notified about how they will be informed about the interview date and time. The expectation that students will treat this as though it were an actual job interview needs to be highlighted and that they will receive feedback on all aspects of the process including their punctuality, appearance and performance.

Review of Application Forms

The application forms will be reviewed by the facilitators acting as interviewers as they will be providing the feedback on the application forms. There is no formal shortlisting process and all students will be invited to attend for an interview. However, if the application form would not have been shortlisted in real life, this will need to be raised with the student and the reasons why given at the post-interview feedback. This is an area that may be adapted so that a shortlisting process does take place and the unsuccessful students would need to receive feedback at this point. Bear in mind though that students would then miss out on the interview experience.

The students will then be invited to attend the interview, formally in a letter or less formally by email or simply a list of interviewees with date, time, room to report to and the name of the staff who will act as the interviewers.

The Interview Day

The time allowed for each interview is 30 minutes in total, with 20 minutes for the actual interview and 10 minutes for discussion between facilitators and feedback to the student.

If requested, the student will need to sign in at the designated place. This can be checked after the exercise to see if the student followed the instructions.

The student will be invited in to the office/classroom and introduced to the interviewers. Between six and eight questions will be asked by the interviewers, who will take turns to ask the questions and document the answers. Following the interviewers' questions, the student will be provided with the opportunity to ask any questions. At the end of the interview, the student will be asked to wait outside. The interviewers will complete the scoring sheet. The student will be invited back; at this stage the interviewers can state that they are 'out of role' and the students can 'relax'. The student will be asked to provide an impression of their performance. Feedback is then provided on punctuality, initial impressions and appearance, performance at interview and any paperwork that was provided by the student, for example, a professional portfolio. Performance at interview will include their ability to answer questions and the quality of their answers. The application form will be reviewed. The outcome of the interview will be told to the student and the scoring sheet used will be given to the student.

Feedback needs to be provided constructively, however, some students may find it difficult to accept comments about their performance and their appearance, especially if they feel that it is suitable for interview.

If provided, the student will need to be encouraged to complete the post-interview review sheet.

Some Common Issues from the Interview

Appearance: students need to ensure that they think about the image they wish to project and the balance between fashionable and professional. It is important that aspects of the appearance do not distract the interviewers from what is actually being said by the student. It may be necessary to discuss obvious body piercings and their impact in a professional context.

Shaking hands: students often feel uncomfortable about shaking hands, however, it is a significant part of the interview process and contributes to the initial assessment made by interviewers (Stewart et al., 2008). The study by Stewart et al. (2008: 1145) concludes that 'the interviewers can obtain important information about employee traits through the ... handshake'. They also suggest that women can improve their initial evaluations by learning to shake hands positively and with a firm grip. An Internet search will provide a huge number of listings providing advice on how to shake hands effectively.

Answering questions: students need to ensure that they are able to sell themselves effectively and identify their qualities which demonstrate that they are ready for the post of qualified healthcare practitioner. Students will discuss the practical and interpersonal skills that they have developed during placements but often neglect to demonstrate the knowledge and academic skills that they developed during the theoretical component of the course. When answering questions, students need to support their answers with examples. Common errors include brief answers or over-long answers, not answering the question, or providing a pre-prepared answer that may not address the question.

Background knowledge: Students also need to demonstrate knowledge of the Trust for which they are applying (if this was identified as part of the simulation) and be able to demonstrate how their particular skills and attributes fit into the ethos and ways of working within the Trust. The students also need to demonstrate knowledge of current issues, both locally and nationally, and be aware of the significance of these issues to them as newly qualified healthcare practitioners.

SAMPLE JOB ADVERT

Band 5 Healthcare Practitioner

City X – General Medical Ward – XXXXXX NHS Trust

Salary: £21,176 – £27, 534

Hours per week: 37.5 Internal rotation

(Continued)

(Continued)

Job Type: Permanent

Reference: AB12345

An exciting opportunity has arisen for a newly qualified practitioner to join our dynamic, forward-thinking team.

Our busy 24-bedded ward provides a wide range of services for XXXXXXX. We have strong multidisciplinary team links to ensure we provide care of the highest quality.

We are a well-staffed area with a strong commitment to encouraging our team in their professional, academic and personal development. We will facilitate the development of your skills in a wide range of clinical areas, leadership and management. You will have the ongoing support of our practice development nurse, who ensures staff have the opportunities they need to provide high quality care and to develop their personal career pathway.

We offer a welcoming environment in which to work, and you will receive preceptorship, an orientation and development programme tailored to your needs, and regular appraisals.

Interested? Why not see if we can offer what you are looking for?

The Trust reserves the right to close this vacancy early if a large number of applications are received. Therefore, we encourage early applications to ensure consideration for this post.

If you are successful and shortlisted for interview for this post you will be contacted by EMAIL within 2–3 weeks of the closing date. Therefore, please ensure that you check your email account regularly as all information, including interview dates and times, will be sent only to your account.

We are committed to flexible working and equal opportunities. Posts may be subject to a CRB check. We operate a non-smoking policy.

When applying for this post it is essential that you read the Job Description and Person Specification and use the 'supporting information' space to demonstrate how your skills, knowledge and experience meet the requirements of the person specification. PLEASE NOTE: Only those candidates who clearly demonstrate how they meet the person specification will be shortlisted for this job.

For further details please contact:

Closing Date:

AN EXAMPLE OF A LETTER INVITING STUDENTS TO INTERVIEW

Vacancy Reference: XXX

DATE

Strictly Private & Confidential

ADDRESS

Dear XXX

Re: **JOB POST**

(Continued)

(Continued)

Thank you for your recent application for the above post. I am pleased to be able to invite you for interview at (TIME) on (DATE). Please report to Reception at ADDRESS.

The interviewers will be NAME and POST.

I would be grateful if you could confirm your attendance by emailing ADDRESS. Should you be unable to attend, your reasons would be appreciated, to enable the continual assessment of employability skills strategy.

Please do not hesitate to contact me if you would like any further information.

I look forward to hearing from you soon.

Yours sincerely,

NAME

TITLE

SAMPLE QUESTIONS AND SCORING SHEET

Table 17.1

Question Number	Question	Score
1	Why do you want to work for this xxx Unit?	
2	You have been a student at University for three years. What theoretical and practical skills have you learnt that will be of value to the job you are applying for?	
3	The issue of (current topical issue) within the nursing profession is currently being debated – what is your view and why?	
4	Which personal characteristics are your greatest assets?	
5	Which personal characteristics cause you the most difficulty?	
6	What can you offer this xxx Unit?	
7	Please give an example of a particularly difficult management situation and how you addressed the problem	
8	Why do you believe you are the best person for this job?	
9	Where do you see yourself in five years' time?	

Scoring system

5	Excellent
4	Above average
2	Average
1	Shows potential
X	Does not meet requirement

REFERENCES

Association of Graduate Careers Advisory Services (2010) *Home page*. Available on: http://www.agcas.org.uk/ [accessed 7 February 2011].

Barrick, M., Swidley, B. and Stewart, G. (2010) 'Initial evaluations in the interview: relationships with subsequent interviewer evaluations and employment offers', *Journal of Applied Psychology*, 95 (6): 1163–72.

Johnstone, I. and Willis, J. (eds) (2010) *What Do Graduates Do?* Manchester: HECSU/AGCAS.

Littleford, D., Halstead, J. and Mulraine, C. (2004) *Career Skills: Opening Doors into the Job Market*. Basingstoke: Palgrave Macmillan.

Maurer, T., Solamon, J., Andrews, K. and Troxtel, D. (2001) 'Interviewee coaching, preparation strategies, and response strategies in relation to performance in situational employment interviews', *Journal of Applied Psychology*, 86 (4): 709–17.

Morton-Holmes, I. (2009) *Interview Tips: Interview Questions*. Graduate Prospects Ltd. Available on: http://www.prospects.ac.uk/interview_questions.htm (Prospects website) [accessed 7 February 2011].

NHS Jobs (2009) NHS website. Available on: http://www.jobs.nhs.uk/ [accessed 8 February 2011].

Nursing Times (2011) *Nursing Times: careers in nursing*. Available on: http://nursingjobs.nursingtimes.net/ [accessed 7 February 2011].

Royal College of Nursing (2010) *Home page*. Available on: http://www.rcn.org.uk/ [accessed 7 February 2011].

Skills for Health (2011) *Identifying Current and Future Employability Skills*. Available on: www.skillsforhealth.org.uk/developing-your-organisations-talent/Employability-Skills-Matrix.aspx [accessed 8 February 2011].

Stewart, G., Dustin, S., Barrick, M. and Darnold, T. (2008) 'Exploring the handshake in employment interviews', *Journal of Applied Psychology*, 93 (5): 1139–46.

Yorke, M. and Knight, P.T. (2006) *Embedding Employability into the Curriculum*. York: The Higher Education Academy.

18

BREAKING BAD NEWS/DEALING WITH DIFFICULT CONVERSATIONS

Paul Turner

Aim

The aim of this chapter is to offer practical advice to help the healthcare professional sensitively manage difficult situations when breaking bad news.

Objectives

- To gain an understanding of the importance of this topic in healthcare curricula
- To develop strategies to better deal with the issue of breaking bad news to a patient or relative.

INTRODUCTION

The difficulties of telling another human being something unpleasant or distressing – in modern parlance 'breaking bad news' – have been with us since time immemorial. The ancient Greeks were prone to 'killing the messenger' if displeased with the message (Clemens and Mayer, 1999). Fortunately this practice has long been abandoned but the need for people, and especially healthcare professionals, to be skilled in this area has never lost its importance.

Current healthcare curricula are especially focussed on the healthcare professional gaining effective communication skills, for example, in nursing education we have seen the publication of *Standards for Pre-registration Nursing Education* (Nursing and Midwifery Council (NMC), 2010). This is threaded throughout with the significance of communication skills and specifically states, 'Uses appropriate and relevant communication skills … conveying "unwelcome news"' (Nursing and Midwifery Council (NMC), 2010: 111).

So can we define effective communication? Malloy et al. (2010: 167) point out that, 'Communication in nursing practice is not a simple, naturally occurring process, but rather a complex endeavour'. Professor Bernard Moss, who has taught this subject for over a decade, veers away from offering a definition: 'communication is a far more complex phenomenon than a set of discrete skills' (2008: 3). So perhaps it would be better to discuss the various components that constitute the skill of breaking bad news.

SO WHAT IS 'BAD NEWS' AND WHY IS IT IMPORTANT TO US?

Obviously this chapter is concerned with the healthcare context, but it is worth stating that bad news is not the sole prerogative of healthcare, although it does constitute an extremely important aspect of the healthcare professional's role. Farrell (1999) defined it as the news of life-threatening illness, disability or impending or actual death. This seems somewhat skewed towards the 'terminal' end of bad news. A more concise definition is offered by Buckman (1984) as, new information that drastically and negatively alters the patient's view of his future. An encompassing summing up of the various definitions that we have had over the years is offered by Gallagher et al. (2010: 35): 'information that is perceived to be in some way unwelcome, as news that the recipient would rather not receive, or rather were not true, and which is likely to impact negatively on his/her life'.

As one may expect, much of the work in this area arises from the field of cancer care, from both past (Maguire, 1999a, 1999b) to present (Stajduhar et al., 2010; Langewitz et al., 2010). However, the need for health professionals to have the requisite skills in this area is not confined to the area of cancer alone. Is it easier for a nurse working in the mental health setting to tell a patient they have schizophrenia or will require lifelong medication to control their illness? Or for a speech and language therapist to be involved in breaking the news that a relative who has had a stroke is never going to be able to speak to them again? Although the consequences of these example diagnoses are not life threatening, the effect on the health professional who is breaking the bad news has similarities.

WHO, WHAT, WHERE AND HOW?

First, who should be involved in the process of breaking bad news and to whom should it be given?

THE PATIENT

'Should we tell the patient?' In the past this was much more commonly asked than it is today. Traditionally it fell mainly at the feet of the doctor to make these types of decisions (who are still very much involved in this today (Liénard et al., 2010)). Some doctors in the past felt it right to keep the bad news from the patient, justifying this action as the belief was it may have been damaging to the patient (Oken, 1961). This paternalistic attitude has faded over time and we are in an age of patient choice, inclusion (NHS, 2010) and 'Human Rights'.

So what 'rights' do patients have to be told bad news? It is not clear cut that the European Convention on Human Rights (Council of Europe, 1950) has anything specific to say on this topic. Article 8 of the Convention, 'respect for private and family life', is probably the closest it comes to being relevant. The Human Rights Act (1998) (this Act incorporated the European Convention on Human Rights into domestic law) begins to offer more relevance; as Article 10, 'freedom of expression', states, 'This right shall include freedom to ... receive and impart information ...'. Couple this with the Sixth Principle of the Data Protection Act (1998), the 'Rights of Data Subjects', who have the right to have access to their personal data, then here are the foundations in law upon which we can base our decisions and can confidently state that patients do have the 'right' to be told.

However, should we have to rely on a legal stance to 'force' us to involve the patient? Immanuel Kant posits that, 'respecting human dignity follows from the fact that humans have special capacity to live autonomously ... To make decisions for others, then, is to fail to respect a person's autonomy' (Stewart, 2010: 2). It is a fundamental aspect of nursing care to treat our patients with respect, encompassing all the aspects that this involves, including the patient's autonomy. Thus, not only is there a legal imperative for us to tell the patient, one of the foundations of our nursing practice – to treat the patient with dignity and respect – also requires us to do so.

THE RELATIVES

The first inclination of the healthcare professional may be to involve a partner (married or otherwise), or if there is no partner, then a sibling or child (depending on considerations of age). However, from the preceding discourse on patients' autonomy, we should first ask the patient who *they* want to be informed/involved. Families are complex social structures and, although many follow our conventional understanding of what a family consists of, all too often the healthcare professional can be caught out by preconceived notions and assumptions with regard to individual families. There is no substitute for the good practice of getting to know not only the patient, but also the patient's family. A good rapport formed early on with family members will potentially head off some problems later when bad news may need to be broken.

THE HEALTHCARE PROFESSIONAL

Breaking bad news is best done via a collaboration of professionals. This section will concentrate on the healthcare professional's role in this collaborative effort, bearing in mind that they play the pivotal role. In the majority of cases, the healthcare professional will have had the closest therapeutic relationship with the patient and relatives. Recent studies suggest that concentrating on that aspect alone provides only a limited view of the experience by the patient (Randall and Wearn, 2005; Tobin and Begley, 2008). Healthcare professionals have a role to play in enhancing and clarifying explanations (possibly including unravelling complex medical terminology for the patient and relatives), answering questions, clearing up misunderstandings and providing ongoing support (Reinke et al., 2010). The process of breaking bad news occurs at all points in the inpatient pathway – from diagnosis, through treatment and rehabilitation, to death (Warnock, 2010).

WHAT SHOULD BE SAID?

There is some evidence to suggest that giving a warning that bad news is on the way may help (Maynard, 1997). This avoids the possibility of the bad news being blurted out, perhaps because of nervousness or inexperience on the part of the heath practitioner. A warning allows the psychological preparation of the patient to begin. It is a method advocated in the SPIKES protocol (Baile et al., 2000; see also Table 18.1), a good explanation of which is to be found in Buckman (2005). An example of a such a warning is, 'Mr Smith, I have some bad news for you', as an opener to the conversation.

General points to keep in mind include the following. First, avoid hiding behind jargon, for example, why say 'the malignancy has metastasised' when you could say 'the cancer has spread'? If you need to communicate the fact that someone has died, then the message must be clear and unambiguous. Do not use phrases such as, 'passed away' (Frost et al., 2010); the appropriate approach has to be along the lines of, 'I'm extremely sorry to have to tell you that your father has died'. Whatever the news you have just relayed, you then need to stop talking and give the person time to react. A range of reactions can occur at this point and one of the best options for the health practitioner is to stay silent and allow the person time to start processing the information. Expressions of empathy and physical contact can play a part here; a slight increase in physical closeness or a touch on the hand can be effective in conveying that empathetic connection (Stajduhar et al., 2010). Continue once the person is ready to proceed, but break the information into small chunks and stop periodically to check the patient's understanding (National Council for Hospices and Specialist Palliative Care Services, 2003).

Table 18.1   The SPIKES Protocol

S = Setting	Privacy. Involve significant others. Sit down. Look attentive and calm. Listening skills. Availability
P = Perception (i.e. patient's perception of the current situation)	Note different ways of asking; note patient's vocabulary and comprehension; also note denial, if present
I = Invitation (Aim to get a clear invitation from the patient to share information)	Different ways of asking (e.g. 'Are you the kind of person who prefers to know all the details about what is going on?'). Accept the patient's right not to know too
K = Knowledge (imparting information)	Before you break bad news, give your patient a warning that bad news is coming
	Aligning: start at a place compatible with the patient's current comprehension. Convey information in small chunks. Use plain English not technical or scientific language. Acknowledge all patient's responses and tailor delivery of information appropriately to a patient's responses
E = Empathy	Acknowledge emotions and their origins – both the patient's and your own – and respond appropriately. Explore, validate and empathise with their emotional responses
S = Strategy and Summary	Make a plan via explanation and collaboration. Summarise main areas. Any questions for now? Present a clear plan of the next steps

Source: Baile et al. (2000)

Do not fall into the trap of saying, 'I know how you feel', in an attempt to make an empathetic connection with the recipient of the bad news. You do not. Even if you have experienced loss, encountered the same situation or even been given the same diagnosis, you cannot interpret whether the individual before you is feeling the same way you did.

Another potential minefield to navigate is if the person comes back with the 'Why?' questions: 'Why has this happened to such a nice person?', 'Why has God allowed this to happen?' and/or variations of this response. It is not for you to bring your own 'agenda' into play here (Moss, 2008). It is probably best to maintain the silence or give a neutral response along the lines of, 'I'm sorry I have no answer to that'.

An unhurried approach cannot be overemphasised. Stajduhar's et al.'s study found that, 'Direct eye contact, active listening techniques, sitting down rather than standing and not appearing hurried in their speech or body language were examples that participants gave of the ways clinicians demonstrated they had "all the time in the world"' (2010: 2042).

Once the talking has come to its natural conclusion, remember the importance of written communication. People can only take in so much information at the best of times but, in stressful situations such as when hearing bad news, this is exacerbated. Some of the many local variations in the form that written information can take in today's health service include:

- Information leaflets available in multiple languages
- References to websites offering information on particular health topics and/or diseases
- Names and addresses of specialist care services
- Contact details for self-help groups.

Possible sources of follow-up information are numerous and varied; the healthcare professional can assist by directing the patient/relatives appropriately.

WHERE AND HOW SHOULD BAD NEWS BE BROKEN?

Whenever possible, time should be spent in preparation prior to the event. Staff members need to gather information, ensure they are clear in the message that needs to be delivered, have key personnel available and, ideally, control the environment where the news is broken. The team will face questions and should be prepared to answer them. Jurkovich et al. (2000), in a survey of families who had faced sudden bereavement, found that the most important aspects of giving bad news were: the attitude of the news-giver, combined with clarity of the message, and the time, privacy, and knowledge to answer questions. Thus, the importance of having a private room available for this purpose cannot be under-estimated. Frost et al. (2010) make the point that the staff involved in this process should switch off pagers and mobile phones before entering the room. This is such a simple yet vital detail but, in an age where these devices are so ubiquitous, it is easy to forget; similarly, if there is a landline in the room to be used, set this to 'divert'. Pagers and phones going off in the middle of telling someone their loved one has died would surely add to their distress.

Arrange the room so there is adequate seating. Again a simple point, but people should be sat down and on the same level as each other. Such orchestration of the room setup is beneficial. Standing over someone or perching on the edge of a desk can be intimidating and may give impression that you are more likely to leave, while being sat with someone indicates quite the opposite – that you do have time for them and you are not about to leave. Have a box of tissues available – tears are likely.

Inform other members of the team about what is happening; you do not want other staff members coming into the room unexpectedly. It is highly embarrassing for them and distressing for everyone else.

POINTS TO NOTE

Breaking bad news in a professional and sensitive manner is one of the most important roles of the healthcare professional. When teaching or performing this skill, the importance of preparation cannot be overemphasised and simple things can make a big difference:

- Prepare yourself and your environment
- Consider the use of a warning that bad news is on the way
- Avoid jargon
- Be clear and unambiguous in your message
- Establish a therapeutic connection
- Never state, 'I know how you feel'
- Never rush.

CONCLUSION

> Though it be honest, it is never good to bring bad news (*Antony and Cleopatra*, Act 2, Scene 5, Shakespeare, 1606)

This is a difficult but necessary part of the health professional's role. Done well, it can leave the patient (if it is a non-fatal situation) and their relatives with a benign impression of the person(s) breaking the news. Done badly, it can exacerbate an already difficult situation and fracture that therapeutic relationship health professionals strive to achieve.

To help the health professional in managing and improving their practice there is now a wealth of literature and research available on this topic. This chapter has set out an introduction to the topic of breaking bad news; there is much to further investigate if the reader wishes to do so. We would particularly recommend the SPIKES strategy (Buckman, 2005). As with most things, 'practice makes perfect', and exploring and practising this skill via the medium of simulation can help participants acquire the repertoire of skills and knowledge which will aid them in better managing these fraught circumstances.

Learning Objectives

At the end of the session the student should be able to:

- Discuss the management of a deteriorating patient
- List the members of the multidisciplinary team who may be involved in the patient's care
- Devise a strategy of care for a deceased patient
- Suggest approaches for communicating with relatives at different stages of breaking bad news.

SIMULATION SCENARIO

Setting and Procedure

This exercise is to be carried out in the classroom environment as group work.

- Students to be in groups of five to six; this is a difficult subject and mutual support is inherent in arranging students into groups of these numbers rather than smaller groups
- Desks to be at the side of the room, students to be sat facing each other
- The facilitator will first read out the handover and background information for Eric Preston to the whole group
- The facilitator will then give the instructions presented in 'Task 1' for the groups to discuss
- After five minutes the facilitator will ask for feedback from the groups and lead discussion on the issues raised
- This process will be repeated until all three stages of the scenario have been presented, discussed and fed back.

Handover Information

Eric Preston, 78. End stage Carcinoma of the lung with metastasies in the liver

Also has chest infection

Not For Resuscitation (DNR)

Mr Preston is now requiring all care and is drifting in and out of consciousness

Currently being nursed on an air mattress; four-hourly turns

Requiring regular suction and oral care

Intravenous fluids running 1 litre over 12

Diamorphine pump running 1:24 due at 15.00 hours

Family aware of poor prognosis – Next of kin details supplied.

Task 1

You have been made aware that the condition of Eric Preston is deteriorating.

His family, with whom you have built up a good relationship, are currently not on the ward.

In your groups, plan the actions that you would take as a trained nurse at the point at which you are informed of the change in condition. Think in detail as to what you would say and do to anyone you needed to speak to.

What other actions would need to be taken?

Feedback 1

All groups feedback as to their actions.

Discussion Points and Possible Actions:

- Check the DNR order for dates/signatures
- Call in the next of kin – how would they phrase this?
- Move the patient to the side room for privacy and dignity

- Monitor the patient – have someone stay with him
- Contact doctor to be available to speak to the relatives.

Task 2

Before the family arrives Mr Preston dies. Now discuss in your groups how you will prepare for the arrival of the family, who you know are on their way to the hospital.
Also discuss how this situation would make you feel. Have you experienced this?

Feedback 2

All groups to feedback their thoughts and actions.

Discussion Points and Possible Actions:

- Do they have someone looking out for relatives?
- Quiet room available to use to speak to relatives?
- Inform medical staff
- Positioning and care given to deceased
- Contact Priest, Rabbi, etc. – religious input
- Bereavement literature
- Inform other staff of the situation
- Clear away equipment
- Care of other patients.

Task 3

Mr Preston's family arrive on the ward. Discuss how you would deal with this situation; the following questions are helpful to prompt discussion:

- What would you say when they first arrive?
- Where would you take them?
- How would you deliver the news that Mr Preston has died?
- What reactions might you get form the family?
- What information would you need to give to the family before they left the ward?

Once you have discussed these issues, *practise actually delivering the news* of the death to each other in your group. This may feel strange and 'unreal', but it may be the only experience you get to do this before you have to do it in the real world.

Feedback 3

Student feedback and discussion around the points given in the task above, possibly linking to issues below:

- Asking family to come into office/day room/relatives' room
- How do you tell someone a family member has died? Have any students seen this done in practice – is there a right way of doing this?

- Facilitators may wish to share their own experiences of this situation
- Debrief for any students on the ward
- Offering comfort, body language, tea and coffee, viewing the body. Trust policy will dictate which literature you will be able to hand to relatives
- Use of language – the word 'died' rather than 'passed away' or 'moved on'
- What are we worried about? Hysterics, aggression, denial? Remember in this situation the nurse has a good relationship with the family and this is an expected death. Does this make a difference?
- Procedure: the doctor has to be contacted to certify the death, how do the family collect the death certificate – trust procedures.

USEFUL RESOURCES

The Breaking Bad News website is helpful for further discussion of this element of a healthcare professional's role; see http://www.breakingbadnews.co.uk/.

In most trusts, relatives are advised to contact the bereavement service after 10.00 a.m. the following day to make an appointment. At this meeting the bereavement staff will provide the Medical Certificate of Cause of Death, explain the procedures for registration of death and return any remaining property.

Once relatives inform their chosen funeral directors of the death, the funeral directors will deal directly with bereavement services to arrange collection of the body.

Healthcare professionals will have to explain this procedure to relatives and supply the trust leaflet reinforcing this advice.

Relatives can view the body on the ward at the time of death, further viewings at later times are often organised by bereavement services. A member of the ward staff will need to support this by accompanying the relatives at these viewings.

REFERENCES

Baile, W.F., Buckman, R., Lenzi, R., Glober, G., Beale, E.A. and Kudelka, A.P. (2000) 'SPIKES – A six step protocol for delivering bad news: application to the patient with cancer', *The Oncologist*, 5 (4): 302–11.

Buckman, R. (1984) *I Don't Know What to Say – How to Help and Support Someone Who is Dying*. London: Papermac.

Buckman, R.A. (2005) 'Breaking bad news: the S-P-I-K-E-S strategy', *Community Oncology*, 2 (2): 138–42.

Clemens, J. and Mayer, D.F. (1999) *The Classic Touch: Lessons in Leadership from Homer to Hemingway*. Lincolnwood: Contemporary Books.

Council of Europe (1950) *European Convention on Human Rights*. Rome: Council of Europe.

Data Protection Act (1998) London: HMSO.

Farrell, M. (1999) 'The challenge of breaking bad news', *Intensive and Critical Care Nursing*, 15 (2): 101–110.

Frost, P.J., Leadbeatter, S. and Wise, M.P. (2010) 'Managing sudden death in hospital', *BMJ*, 340: 1024–8.

Gallagher, A., Arber, A., Chaplin, R. and Quirk, A. (2010) 'Service users' experience of receiving bad news about their mental health', *Journal of Mental Health*, 19 (1): 34–42.

Human Rights Act (1998) London: HMSO.

Jurkovich, G.J., Pierce, B., Pananen, L. and Rivara, F.P. (2000) 'Giving bad news: the family perspective', *The Journal of Trauma*, 48 (5): 865–73.

Langewitz, W., Heydrich, L., Nübling, M., Szirt, L., Weber, H. and Grossman, P. (2010) 'Swiss cancer league communication skills training programme for oncology nurses: an evaluation', *Journal of Advanced Nursing*, 66 (10): 2266–77.

Liénard, A., Merckaert, I., Libert, Y., Bragard, I., Delvaux, N., Etienne, A-M,. Marchal, S., Meunier, J., Reynaert, C., Slachmuylder, J.-L. and Razavi, D. (2010) 'Is it possible to improve residents breaking bad news skills? A randomised study assessing the efficacy of a communication skills training program', *British Journal of Cancer*, 102: 171–7.

Maguire, P. (1999a) 'Improving communication with cancer patients', *European Journal of Cancer*, 35 (10): 1415–22.

Maguire, P. (1999b) 'Improving communication with cancer patients', *European Journal of Cancer*, 35 (14): 2058–65.

Malloy, P., Virani, R., Kelly, K. and Munévar, C. (2010) 'Beyond bad news: communication skills of nurses in palliative care', *Journal of Hospice & Palliative Nursing*, 12 (3): 166–74.

Maynard, D.W. (1997) 'How to tell patients bad news: the strategy of "forecasting"', *Cleveland Clinical Journal of Medicine*, 64 (4): 181–2.

Moss, B. (2008) *Communication Skills for Health and Social Care*. London: Sage.

National Council for Hospices and Specialist Palliative Care Services (2003) *Breaking Bad News ... Regional Guidelines*. Belfast: Department of Health, Social Services and Public Safety.

National Health Service (NHS) (2010) *The NHS Constitution*. London: NHS.

Nursing and Midwifery Council (NMC) (2010) *Standard for Pre-Registration Nursing Education*. London: NMC.

Oken, D. (1961) 'What to tell cancer patients: a study of medical attitudes', *Journal of the American Medical Association*, 175: 1120–8.

Randall, T. and Wearn, A. (2005) 'Receiving bad news: patients with haematological cancer reflect on their experiences', *Palliative Medicine*, 19: 594–601.

Reinke, L.F., Shannon, S.E., Engelberg, R.A., Young, J.P. and Randall Curtiss, J. (2010) 'Supporting hope and prognostic information: nurses' perspectives on their role when patients have life-limiting prognoses', *Journal of Pain and Symptom Management*, 39 (6): 982–92.

Stajduhar, K.I., Thorne, S.E., McGuinness, L. and Kim-Sing, C. (2010) 'Patient perceptions of helpful communication in the context of advanced cancer', *Journal of Clinical Nursing*, 19: 2039–47.

Stewart, R.S. (2010) 'Telling patients the truth', *The Online Journal of Heath Ethics*, 6 (1): 1–10.

Tobin, G. and Begley, C. (2008) 'Receiving bad news. A phenomenological exploration of the lived experience of receiving a cancer diagnosis', *Cancer Nursing*, 31 (5): E31–E39.

Warnock, C., Tod, A., Foster, J. and Soreny, C. (2010) 'Breaking bad news in inpatient clinical settings: role of the nurse', *Journal of Advanced Nursing*, 66 (7): 1543–55.

19

INCIDENT REPORTING

Tim Badger

Aim

The aim of this chapter is to describe a simulated learning activity through which healthcare students learn about incident reporting.

Objectives

- To identify the principles of incident reporting
- To explain the role of incident reporting in promoting patient safety, with examples of good practice
- To explore reasons why incidents may not be reported.

INTRODUCTION

Incident reporting is the process by which adverse events in healthcare are documented, analysed and used for learning to improve patient safety and practice. In the healthcare situation an incident means any 'event or circumstance that could have resulted, or did result, in unnecessary damage, loss or harm such as physical or mental injury to a patient, staff, visitors or members of the public' (National Reporting and Learning Service 2010a: 8). This definition makes it clear that incidents are defined not only as events which happened but also 'near misses'. The severity of an event, or the potential severity of a near miss, does not determine whether it is an incident. However, there is an additional definition for a serious incident – serious incidents include ones which result in unexpected or avoidable death, serious harm, allegations of abuse, threaten the delivery of healthcare service, produce adverse media reports or raise public concern, or are listed as 'never events' by the National Reporting and Learning Service (2010b). The simulation described in this chapter will focus on the general definition of an incident as one that all healthcare practitioners will need to report.

The standards of conduct, performance and ethics of healthcare regulators (Health Professions Council (HPC), 2008; Nursing and Midwifery Council (NMC), 2008) identify the importance of maintaining safety, managing risk, and keeping clear and accurate records, which are all key elements of incident reporting. These requirements make incident reporting an essential skill for maintaining patient safety which healthcare students must learn as they prepare for registration. Although the onus for reporting patient safety incidents lies with the registered professional, from their first practical experience students may be involved in reporting incidents involving personal injury or loss of personal belongings.

BACKGROUND TO INCIDENT REPORTING

Accounts of incident reporting all recognise the importance of first responding promptly to the incident that is ensuring prompt treatment for anyone who has actually been injured. When it comes to reporting and recording the incident, Power (2010) identifies that the subsequent advice varies – some focusing on defensive approaches of not apologising or admitting liability to avoid claims. By contrast Siviter (2008) points out the role of incident reporting in raising and escalating concerns, stating that where patients are at risk which the individual practitioner cannot personally resolve, those concerns must be reported in writing as an incident report. Incident reporting thus has several purposes:

- To enable incidents which have caused harm to be investigated and documented
- To enable lessons to be learnt from incidents, including near misses, to prevent recurrence and improve patient safety
- To identify trends in incidents and patient safety risks
- To ensure legal and NHS governance requirements are met.

Incident reporting will normally use a standard form requiring details of the date, time and location of the incident; the name, address, age and gender of affected persons; whether the affected person was a member of staff, patient or visitor; details of the injury or dangerous occurrence; and actions taken.

Once a report is completed it must be passed to whoever has designated responsibility for investigating incidents. Within the National Health Service, incident report (IR1) forms are commonly completed as an online form, as this promotes prompt transmission of the report to the person responsible for investigating the incident. A second form (IR2) is used to record the investigation of the incident.

Where an injured person is an employee this investigation must take account of statutory responsibilities regarding the reporting of workplace injuries as required by Reporting of Injuries, Diseases and Dangerous Occurrences Regulations 1995 (RIDDOR).

The completing of incident reports should be regarded as an example of record keeping. Therefore, completion of an incident report should follow the principles of good record keeping. These principles include that records 'should be accurate and recorded in such a way that the meaning is clear ... (and) should be factual and not include unnecessary abbreviations, jargon, meaningless phrases or irrelevant speculation' (Nursing and Midwifery Council, 2009: 4). The incident report should be completed as near to the time of the incident as possible. Although it should be obvious, it is an important principle that providing treatment to the injured person takes priority over report writing.

Separate forms should be completed for each person directly affected by the incident, therefore two incident reports would be required where two patients both fell on the same patch of wet floor. The member of staff who is the first to know about the incident should usually complete the incident form. Thus if a student hurts their back during patient handling, the student should complete the incident report. Although the student may complete the report in this situation, their supervisor still has a professional duty and employment responsibilities to ensure the report is completed and should check the report's accuracy and completeness before it is submitted.

CURRENT THEORY AND GOOD PRACTICE IN INCIDENT REPORTING

Employers have a clearly identified legal obligation towards their staff (which includes placement students and volunteers). This chapter will not discuss in detail the requirements of health and safety legislation, however, the reporting of some incidents is required by the Reporting of Injuries, Diseases and Dangerous Occurrences Regulations 1995 (RIDDOR). RIDDOR is a legal requirement on employers and persons in charge of the workplace, which enables risk assessment and serious accident investigation by the Health and Safety Executive (HSE) and local authorities. This leads to advice to employers on the reduction of workplace injury and ill health. RIDDOR requirements for reporting include incidents resulting in death, major injury, absence from work over three days, specified diseases, dangerous occurrences and gas incidents.

In the healthcare setting incidents do not occur to staff alone but also affect patients and visitors. The legal aspects of the two may differ; for example, injury to a member of staff during patient handling may require RIDDOR reporting, while an injury to a patient during the same procedure would not. Local incident reporting policies may differentiate between incidents affecting patient safety and those which do not. These are sometimes termed clinical and non-clinical incidents, although it may seem confusing that a nurse sustaining a needle-stick injury while preparing an injection would be classed as a non-clinical injury. Fortunately for practitioners, the reporting procedure using an NHS IR1 form is the same for all incidents whether affecting patients, visitors or staff.

Although legal liability for patients is not covered by health and safety at work legislation, the legal duty of care towards patients is equally strong. Florence Nightingale's well-known maxim that 'the hospital should do the sick no harm' is a useful reminder of this, and the establishment of the National Patient Safety Agency in 2001 emphasises that it remains a priority. Incident reporting is one of the seven steps to patient safety described by the National Patient Safety Agency (2004). These steps are:

1 Build a safety culture, by creating an open and fair culture;
2 Lead and support staff to establish a clear and strong focus on patient safety;
3 Integrate your risk management activity, by developing systems and processes to manage risks and identify and assess things that could go wrong;
4 Promote reporting, by ensuring staff can easily report incidents;
5 Involve and communicate with patients and the public, by developing ways to communicate openly with and listen to patients;
6 Learn and share safety lessons, encouraging staff to use root cause analysis to learn how and why incidents happen;
7 Implement solutions to prevent harm, by embedding lessons through changes to practice.

These steps focus more on the role of healthcare managers rather than that of practitioners, which may explain Cross et al.'s (2007) finding that managers have a more positive view of incident reporting than clinical staff, despite the potential for clinical staff to use incident reporting to improve care. The issues of an open and fair culture to promote reporting and the processes for reporting incidents are clearly relevant to healthcare students, and are discussed later in this chapter.

Learning lessons to improve safety is a key aim of incident reporting. The NHS Litigation Authority states:

> Incident reporting provides an opportunity for adverse events to be documented, analysed and used for learning and improvements in practice. Incident reporting is a key requirement for NHS organisations in efforts to improve patient safety and should be seen as an important way for organisations to manage performance and assure staff, patients and the public that systems for managing risk are robust and effective. (2010: 99)

This focus of incident reporting on patient safety remains the same, whether or not the incident is classed as serious. Some serious incidents are considered to be 'never events', which are serious, preventable patient safety incidents which should not occur if the available preventative measures have been implemented (National Reporting and Learning Service, 2010b). One of these is wrong route administration of chemotherapy: the Department of Health (2008) identified that there had been at least 55 incidents recorded worldwide where death or paralysis had occurred following the injection of the drug vincristine intrathecally (into the spinal fluid) rather than intravenously. Donaldson (2003) had previously pointed out that the known cases were only those which had been reported in journals or otherwise made public rather than the true incidence, and that systems could be put in place to prevent recurrence.

Cross et al. (2007) examined the reporting culture of why people do or do not report incidents. They identified six categories for non-reporting:

- Individual attitude to mistakes: staff members who think incidents are solely in their control are unlikely to report them
- Management attitude to mistakes: regarding incidents as the fault of individuals rather than systems discourages open reporting
- Perceived consequences of 'admitting' to a mistake: staff who expected to be affected professionally or personally will be discouraged from reporting incidents
- Organisational sharing of experience: whether staff perceive an organisational culture in which they feel able or encouraged to share experience
- Organisational response to problems: staff who see little or no evidence of feedback see no point in reporting incidents
- Characteristics of incident reporting systems: unless a system is easy to use, staff are discouraged from reporting incidents.

A just or 'no blame' culture is recommended as one way to encourage reporting incidents to promote learning, to overcome the barrier identified above of perceived personal consequences. This recognises that patient safety incidents are often not the fault of individual practitioners but a result of the systems in which people work. Reason's (2000) Swiss Cheese model for analysing patient safety incidents has been adopted in many National Patient Safety Agency reports. In this model each stage in a procedure is regarded as providing barriers or layers of defence to prevent possible harm. However, each of those barriers has holes (which can be compared to Swiss cheese): when all of the holes are aligned the possible harm reaches the patient and safety is compromised. Figure 19.1 illustrates some of the barriers in preventing medication error, indicating that error may occur at the stages of prescription, dispensing, administration or monitoring.

This model recognises that healthcare systems and procedures are the root cause of many patient safety incidents, rather than individual error or randomness. It should be obvious that where patient safety is compromised by deliberate action this does not apply. Burns (2007) suggests that, although there are clear benefits to a 'no blame' culture in promoting patient safety, often this does not satisfy people who feel their trust in healthcare organisations has been betrayed and want staff to be held to account.

Good practice recommends reporting not just actual incidents which have occurred but also 'near misses', where patient safety was at risk but harm averted. Incident reporting is thus one way in which practitioners may raise or escalate concerns about practice ('whistleblowing'). Bellefontaine (2009) found that the culture of not reporting concerns begins with students who witness poor practice, where they fear

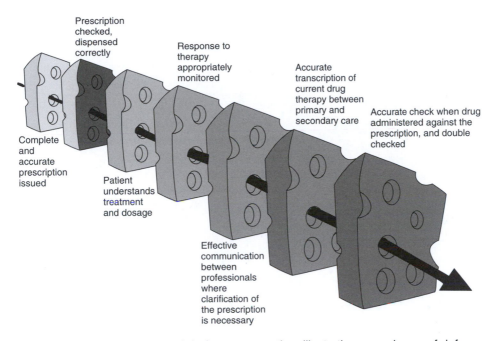

Prescription
checked,
dispensed
correctly

Response to
therapy
appropriately
monitored

Accurate
transcription of
current drug
therapy between
primary and
secondary care

Accurate check when drug
administered against the
prescription, and double
checked

Complete
and
accurate
prescription
issued

Patient
understands
treatment
and dosage

Effective
communication
between
professionals
where
clarification of
the prescription
is necessary

Figure 19.1   Swiss cheese model of error prevention, illustrating some layers of defence
against medication error

Source: Department of Health (2004) *Building a Safer NHS for Patients: Improving Medication Safety*.
London: Department of Health. ©Crown Copyright 2011

retaliation or lack of support from practitioners, or are anxious that they would be labelled as troublesome; they might also have been put off raising concerns by the stress of the procedures involved.

A review by Aygemang and While (2010) identified that medication errors by nurses can be categorised as preparation errors and administration errors. Medication errors include wrong dosage, dose omission, wrong medication or form of medication, wrong patient, wrong time, wrong solvent, labelling errors; administration errors include wrong route or rate of administration. They identified that contributing factors to medication errors can be categorised as personal and organisational factors. Personal factors include policies and procedures, stress and tiredness, and knowledge of medication, while organisation factors may be distractions and interruptions, systems for medication delivery, the quality of prescribing, workloads and the need to multitask, and technology design.

The Department of Health (2004) stated that the true incidence of medication errors is unknown, as many go unnoticed or unreported if no serious harm occurs to the patient. They compared the reporting of errors to an iceberg (seven-eighths of which is underwater): their illustration (see Figure 19.2) shows that most errors causing actual harm are reported, while most near-misses with potential to cause harm, errors considered insignificant, and potential and unnoticed actual errors go unreported.

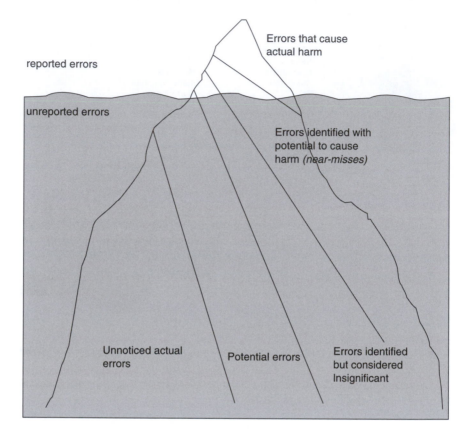

Figure 19.2   The iceberg of medication errors

Source: Department of Health (2004) *Building a Safer NHS for Patients: Improving Medication Safety*. London: Department of Health. ©Crown Copyright 2011

As an example of the effects of a positive reporting culture, Bonner and Wellman (2010) studied post-incident review of aggression and violence in an acute mental health unit. They discussed that although serious incidents are reported and reviewed, less serious incidents – for example, where no injury occurred or prolonged restrain was not required – are not routinely reviewed, with the result that post-incident support is often missed. They found that a simple reporting system gave participants an opportunity to review incidents and learn from them, and helped minimise the psychological impact of aggression. In showcasing examples of good practice the National Reporting and Learning Service (2008) described a ward where the practice was not in line with the local policy for reporting of accidents and incidents, and where staff were confused about when incident reports should be completed. Following education about the management of slips, trips and falls more incident reports were completed; as a result changes were made to footwear, cleaning and flooring.

POINTS TO NOTE

Healthcare providers have their own policies for reporting untoward incidents, and familiarity with local policies and procedures is essential for good practice and facilitating this simulation. For National Health Service (NHS) Trusts these are often available through the individual organisation's Freedom of Information Publication Scheme. Independent and voluntary sector organisations will have their own incident reporting policies as required by the Care Quality Commission, however, UK freedom of information legislation only covers public authorities.

CONCLUSION

Incident reporting is a requirement of legal, employment and professional obligations. Within a healthcare organisation, procedures for reporting incidents affecting patients, visitors and staff should be clearly identified. Incident reporting may be seen as a defensive strategy to defend against legal claims, but there is a current emphasis on using incidents as a tool for learning and improving patient safety from the National Learning and Reporting Service (a division of the National Patient Safety Agency), which has identified good practice in achieving this. Although a 'no blame culture' should improve reporting and enable learning from incidents to occur, there is still significant under-reporting of incidents due to fear of punitive action being taken against the staff involved.

Incident Reporting

An Introduction to the Simulation

The purpose of this simulation is for students to discuss whether a clinical event requires an incident report. In this simulation a recently qualified registered practitioner thinks that they have made a medication administration error but, based on their knowledge of the drugs involved, does not think harm will occur to the patient and feels certain they will learn from the error to practise safely in future. The practitioner asks the advice of a senior colleague about what they should do.

Learning Outcomes

By completing this simulation students will be able to:

- Discuss situations when an incident report should be completed
- Explain the reasons for completing an incident report with reference to patient safety and professional standards
- Explain how to report an incident and what information will be required.

SIMULATION SCENARIO

Resources Required

The environment for this simulation should represent an office area on a ward. The following documents should be available to consult:

- A local healthcare provider's policy for reporting untoward incidents: familiarity with this is recommended for facilitating this simulation. For NHS Trusts this policy may be available through the individual organisation's Freedom of Information Publication Scheme
- Nursing and Midwifery Council *Standards for Medicines Management* (2007) and *Record Keeping: Guidance for Nurses and Midwives* (2009)
- British National Formulary.

As an incident report (IR1) would normally be completed online, completion of the report will probably not be practical within the simulation. Where this is possible (and sufficient time is available), the scenario may be extended to make this possible.

Roles of Participants

Table 19.1

Participant 1 (student or facilitator): recently qualified Registered Nurse	You are working on a rehabilitation ward and have performed a drug administration round by yourself as allowed by local policy. You feel under pressure today as the ward has been affected by staff sickness. While preparing to give Mr Green his tablets you were interrupted, and you realise afterwards that you have given him Flucloxacillin 250mg orally rather than Amoxycillin 250mg as prescribed. Mr Green noticed at the time that the tablets looked different but you reassured him that you had just opened a new packet. You mentioned this to the ward doctor who said not to worry as they'd just received laboratory results and were about to change Mr Green's antibiotics anyway and that he was obviously not allergic to penicillin.
	You tell the experienced nurse who is in charge about this, asking how to document this. You recognise that you have made a mistake and have learned from it, but as you have spoken to the doctor you don't think any further action is needed. If the nurse in charge suggests further actions are needed you are afraid of 'getting into trouble' and don't want to be thought unreliable or lacking competence.
Participant 2 (student): experienced Registered Nurse	You are the practitioner in charge today on a rehabilitation ward. A recently qualified Registered Nurse tells you that they have made a drug administration error. You want to make sure that they have responded appropriately to this error in terms of ensuring patient safety, completing an incident report, and informing the patient. If necessary you will need to explain how to report an incident.

Discussion Points and Areas of Consideration for the Facilitator

You will need to ensure the learning outcomes are met by ensuring that patient safety is prioritised, reasons for requiring an incident report are clear, and that the process of incident reporting is explained.

Discussion points should include:

- The role of incident reporting in improving patient safety
- Reasons why incidents may not be reported
- Whether a 'no blame culture' exists and whether one is beneficial
- Causes of medication errors and strategies to prevent them.

REFERENCES

Agyemang, R.E.O. and While, A. (2010) 'Medication errors: types, causes and impact on nursing practice', *British Journal of Nursing*, 19 (6): 380–5.

Bellefontaine, N. (2009) 'Exploring whether student nurses report poor practice they have witnessed on placement', *Nursing Times*, 105 (35): 28–31.

Bonner, G. and Wellman, S. (2010) 'Postincident review of aggression and violence in mental health settings', *Journal of Psychosocial Nursing*, 48 (7): 35–40.

Burns, F. (2007) 'Name of the game is not "no blame"', *Health Services Journal*, 17 (6051): 16–17. Available on: http://www.hsj.co.uk/name-of-the-game-is-not-no-blame/58151 [accessed 26 January 2011].

Cross, S., Whittington, C. and Miller, Z. (2007) *NHS Scotland Incident Reporting Culture*. Glasgow: NHS Quality Improvement Scotland.

Department of Health (DH) (2004) *Building a Safer NHS for Patients: Improving Medication Safety*. London: Department of Health.

Department of Health (DH) (2008) *Updated National Guidance on the Safe Administration of Intrathecal Chemotherapy (HSC 2008/001)*. London: Department of Health.

Donaldson, L. (2003) *Annual Report of the Chief Medical Officer 2002*. London: Department of Health.

Health Professions Council (2008) *Standards of Conduct Performance and Ethics*. London: HPC.

National Patient Safety Agency (NPSA) (2004) *Seven Steps to Patient Safety*. London: National Patient Safety Agency.

National Reporting and Learning Service (2008) *7 Steps to Patient Safety in Mental Health: Good Practice Examples*. London: National Patient Safety Agency.

National Reporting and Learning Service (2010a) *National Framework for Reporting and Learning from Serious Incidents Requiring Investigation*. London: National Patient Safety Agency.

National Reporting and Learning Service (2010b) *Never Events Framework: Update for 2010–11*. London: National Patient Safety Agency.

NHS Litigation Authority (2010) *NHSLA Risk Management Handbook 2010/11*. London: NHS Litigation Authority.

Nursing and Midwifery Council (NMC) (2007) *Standards for Medicine Management*. London: NMC.

Nursing and Midwifery Council (NMC) (2008) *The Code: Standards of Conduct Performance and Ethics for Nurses and Midwives*. London: Nursing and Midwifery Council.

Nursing and Midwifery Council (NMC) (2009) *Record Keeping: Guidance for Nurses and Midwives*. London: Nursing and Midwifery Council.

Power, K. (2010) 'What is involved in incident reporting?', in J. Fowler (ed.), *Staff Nurse Survival Guide*, 2nd edn. London: Quay.

Reason, J. (2000) 'Human error: models and management', *British Medical Journal*, 320: 768–70.

Siviter, B. (2008) *The Newly Qualified Nurse's Handbook*. London: Bailliere Tindall.

20

DISCHARGE PLANNING

Lisa Lawton

Aim

By the end of this chapter you will have gained an insight and overview of the discharge planning process and be able to participate in a discharge planning simulation scenario using an identified case study.

Objectives

- To allow the healthcare professional the ability to develop their knowledge and understanding of an effective discharge planning process
- To support personal development
- Understand the relevance of effective communication skills and multi agency working within the process of discharge planning.

INTRODUCTION

Discharge planning, as the terminology suggests, is the process of planning for discharge. As Shepperd et al. state:

> Discharge planning is the development of an individualised discharge plan for the patient prior to leaving hospital, with the aim of containing costs and improving patient outcomes. Discharge planning should ensure that Patients are discharged from hospital at an appropriate time in their care and that with adequate notice the provision of other services will be organised. (2010: 2)

Discharge should not be seen as an isolated event but a process. It also should be considered that discharging a patient does not always refer to being discharged home but can refer to being discharged from one department/clinical area/level of care to another. The National Assembly for Wales circular 2005/17 (Chandler et al., 2008), Hospital Discharge planning guidance suggests that people being discharged from hospital are entitled to expect and receive a smooth transition from one stage of care to the next.

The Department of Health (2004) believes that up to 80 per cent of discharges are simple and should be carried out by nurses, but ensuring patients get home safely is not always as simple and straightforward as it seems. With the continued drive to ensure efficiency and efficacy, and reductions in length of stay and delays in discharge – alongside the increase in patient choice – the demand for effective discharge planning is ever increasing.

Healthcare professionals are required to develop and improve their discharge planning skills in order to meet this demand. The necessary skills to develop include communication, effective assessment and evaluation of needs, as well as the ability to work within a multidisciplinary arena.

By implementing effective and efficient discharge it not only improves patient or client throughput, but also becomes cost efficient as it minimises length of stay, reduces the risk of emergency re-admission and reduces the risk of infection – which, in turn, limits potential further treatment. A lack of coordinated and person-centred planning for discharge can lead to poor outcomes and possible risk for patients with regard to their health and safety, which could lead to re-admission to hospital (Chandler et al., 2008).

Effective discharge planning should be a multi-agency, multi-professional activity to which all healthcare professionals make a contribution. Discharge planning is a 'non-technical' skill and for many healthcare professionals it is not seen as essential. However, according to Rennie (2009), non-technical skills such as communication and team working are as essential and valued in nursing as the more traditional tangible fundamental clinical skills. Carroll and Dowling (2007) concur when they suggest that the essential elements for discharge planning are:

- Communication
- Coordination
- Education
- Patient participation
- Collaboration between medical personnel.

Delays in discharge not only have a financial implication but can also lead to dissatisfied patients and relatives, which can lead to a breakdown in the partnership and trust between the healthcare professional and the patient. This is an area that, undoubtably, healthcare providers can continue to improve upon.

To enable healthcare professionals to establish a robust framework safely to discharge patients, it is important that their communication and assessment skills are addressed during their educational programme alongside leadership skills, which are required in order to lead on what can sometimes be a complex discharge plan. When embedding multi-professional working it is suggested that this required educational knowledge and these skills should be delivered in a multi-professional arena.

Discharge planning can be a crucial element to a patient's experience of hospital care and is relevant to all patients, whether they are a planned or an emergency admission. The Department of Health's discharge planning toolkit (2004) was developed to improve hospital discharges and sets out practical advice and a step-by-step guide to improving the process. As the government drives to reduce costs and improve efficiency, however, it must not be forgotten that quality and the wellbeing of the patient should be at the forefront of any activity within the National Health Service.

Discharge planning should start as early as possible and in a planned admission an expected date of discharge (EDD) should be set on admission, or even at a pre-admission clinic if appropriate. To be able to identify an effective EDD it will be necessary to explore with the patient and their carers/family what their needs at discharge will be and whether this can be supported within their current home circumstances and support mechanisms. By identifying a date and time for expected discharge it will enable the patient, family and carers to plan and be aware of the situation. It is important to review progress throughout the patient's stay to ensure that this date is still suitable, realistic and achievable.

At the start of the discharge process, identifying whether a discharge can be categorised as a 'simple discharge' or one with 'complex needs' will aid a smoother transition for the patient. Nationally up to 805 patients fall into the category of simple discharge needs per day (DH, 2003). These patients are usually able to be discharged back to their own place of residence, have simple ongoing care needs and do not require a complex plan of care post discharge. Patients are categorised as having complex needs either because it is not possible to predict the length of stay in hospital or they have multiple care needs at the point of discharge which require detailed assessment, planning and delivery by multi-professionals and multi-agency teams.

What is also required when an expected date of discharge is being identified, is to be clear what medical and social criteria the patient has to meet to enable them to be deemed fit for discharge. In order for a patient to be able to meet the identified criteria it will be necessary for a coordinated approach with an identified leader for the process to run smoothly.

In 2010 the Department of Health issued a comprehensive guide on planning discharge and transfer of patients from hospital and intermediate care. This guide suggests 10 operating principles.

Figure 20.1 identifies a high-level pathway for the discharge and transfer planning process for simple and complex discharges (Department of Health, 2010).

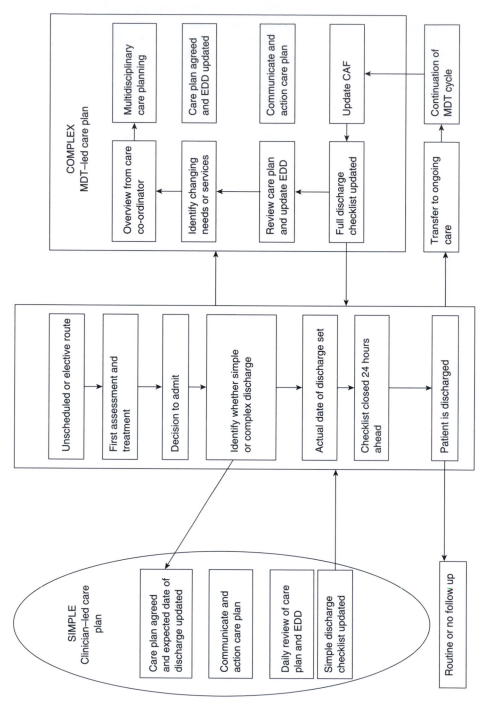

COMPLEX
MDT–led care plan

- Overview from care co-ordinator
- Multidisciplinary care planning
- Identify changing needs or services
- Care plan agreed and EDD updated
- Review care plan and update EDD
- Communicate and action care plan
- Full discharge checklist updated
- Update CAF

- Unscheduled or elective route
- First assessment and treatment
- Decision to admit
- Identify whether simple or complex discharge
- Actual date of discharge set
- Checklist closed 24 hours ahead
- Patient is discharged

SIMPLE
Clinician–led care plan

- Care plan agreed and expected date of discharge updated
- Communicate and action care plan
- Daily review of care plan and EDD
- Simple discharge checklist updated

- Transfer to ongoing care
- Continuation of MDT cycle
- Routine or no follow up

Figure 20.1

HEALTHCARE PROFESSIONALS' ROLE IN DISCHARGE PLANNING

The Royal College of Nursing (2010) highlight the responsibility of nursing staff, in line with their professional Code of Conduct, to act in accordance with the code in:

- Listening to people in their care and respond to their needs and preferences
- Sharing with people in a way they can understand the information they want and need to know about their health and care
- Sharing information with colleagues and keeping them informed. Working effectively as part of a team
- Ensuring that patient consent is gained before intervention
- Acting as advocate for patients (RCN, 2010; NMC, 2008).

Other allied healthcare professional codes concur with the expectations of their practitioners to provide care that puts the needs of the service users at the centre of the decision-making process, alongside respecting and supporting individuals' autonomy. Team working, collaboration and effective communication are all elements that are discussed within all professional codes of conduct (physiotherapists, occupational therapists, etc.). All of these elements are fundamental to ensuring effective and safe discharge for patients/service users.

From the areas highlighted above, the common theme is that of communication – whether it is verbal or written. Covey (2006) suggested that although human beings spend up to three-quarters of their waking time involved in some sort of communication, the majority is by listening. However, this element of communication is not routinely taught to us as a skill.

Communication will take place between healthcare professionals as well as with the patient and their carers. Patient involvement is an essential component to ensuring a smooth discharge. By doing so it enables the patient to feel supported and less confused during the process leaving them feeling less vulnerable or frightened.

As the National Leadership and Innovation Agency for Health's *Passing the Baton* guide to effective discharge states:

> If we build up a rapport with people by being able to empathise with their predicament, fears and concerns and have an understanding about what is of value to them, then we have a significant positive impact upon their experience of our care services. (Chandler et al., 2008: 2.1)

If patients are in agreement and have an understanding of the process and the rationale for the decisions made, they will cooperate with and engage in the process. Accurate record keeping is essential to ensure efficient and effective communication between all members of a discharge team. However, to ensure that all elements of a discharge are completed it is important to identify a lead. As Foust (2007) suggests, although discharge planning is an everyday part of daily nursing practice it can pose significant challenges for nurses.

Timely assessments will assist in the process and for a nurse to be effective in discharge planning they need to ensure they are aware not only of national guidelines such as those of the Department of Health (2004) but also, more importantly, of their local policy and procedures. The National Health Service Institute has developed a series of programmes to reduce waste and take out unnecessary steps, in turn allowing better quality of service. The Productive Series (2009) set up by the National Health Service Institute for Innovation and Improvement, supports healthcare teams to redesign and streamline the way they manage and work. This helps achieve significant and lasting improvements – predominately in the extra time that they give to patients, as well as improving the quality of care delivered, while reducing costs.

The goal is to have every ward, operating theatre and community service operating 'productively' by 2014 and delivering significant benefits for patients, for staff and for the NHS Institute of Innovation and Improvement (2011).

As suggested, there is a series of programmes for the variety of healthcare environments that exist, with the underlying principle being to improve processes and environments to assist nurses and allied health professionals to spend more time on patient care and thereby improve safety and efficiency. Figure 20.2 demonstrates diagrammatically the Productive Series, while the modules within the Productive Ward Programme, which includes a module specifically discussing the admission and discharge processes, are illustrated in Figure 20.3.

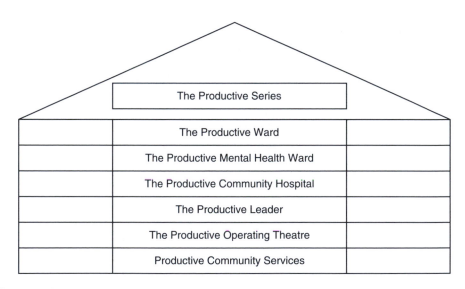

Figure 20.2

Source: Adapted from The Productive Series, NHS Institute of Innovation and Improvement (2009)

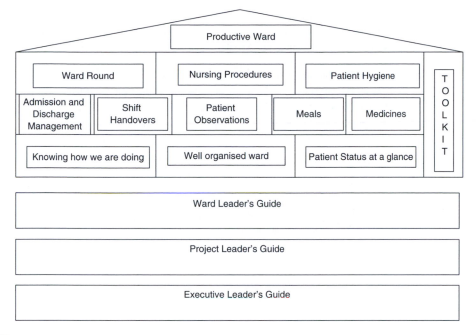

Figure 20.3

Source: Adapted from The Productive Ward Modules (Department of Health, 2009)

Healthcare organisations have either a dedicated discharge planner or team to enable movement of patients throughout the system, whether that is for transferring internally between departments or from service to service – that is, from secondary to primary care, or from secondary to third sector organisations. The overview of the discharge planners enables all patients to access or exit from their required care and interventions.

GOOD PRACTICE EXAMPLES

- Effective and efficient discharge planning starts at admission or, if a planned admission, can start pre-admission. As soon as possible it should be identified what the patient's discharge needs are and identify an expected date of discharge – it can always be changed following reviews. 'Discharge is a process and not an isolated event at the end of the patient's stay' (Department of Health, 2003: 2)
- Identified discharge policy which has a framework for all staff to follow with clear identified roles and responsibilities

- Clear identified timelines and a realistic and achievable Expected Date of Discharge (EDD). To ensure as smooth a process as possible, the Department of Health (2010) suggest various criteria that enable a healthcare professional to set a realistic EDD, using the acronym **START**:

  Set the expected date of discharge according to the patient's condition and diagnosis – This may be more difficult than it sounds as there is no given formula for each diagnosis and each patient is an individual. However, with experience and care pathways being used within the healthcare settings, this can indicate a standard length of stay for the majority of patients with a particular condition or diagnosis.

  Tests and investigations may impact on the EDD as a patient may not be able to be discharged until these have been undertaken; or the date may need to be reviewed if the results are not what was expected.

  Achievable EDD – Base the EDD on how long it should take to get results and assessments, not on how long it actually takes in practice (this enables organisations to identify any constraints)

  Routine – the MDT must set the EDD as part of the routine admissions assessment for every patient, and must regularly review it

  Timely – The EDD must be set within 48 hours of admission to the acute setting, or at pre-admissions assessment, and within four days for community.

TEACHING A SKILL

When considering teaching a skill it is important to identify all the elements of the skill and address each area in turn. Using simulation will enable you to consider each element in a safe environment with students, and enable them to reflect upon their actions to improve if necessary.

As discussed by Benner (1984) it is not sufficient for the learner simply to know a process, it is the demonstration of application that demonstrates competence. Bloom (1956) highlights this in his 'taxonomy of learning'.

Gallagher et al. (2005) suggest that delivering information in a lecture or a classroom rarely develops decision making, attitudes and retrieval; additionally, with limited attention span in the academic setting, information is not retained. Therefore, the traditional classroom setting is not the most suitable arena in which to teach these skills. However, a simulated environment would allow candidates to develop their knowledge base into practice in a safe environment.

TEACHING DISCHARGE PLANNING

To enable future healthcare workers to engage effectively and efficiently in the discharge planning process it is vital that the teaching that occurs within the academic setting of simulation mirrors the processes of the local healthcare settings. Enabling pre-registration students to undertake simulation sessions to develop their knowledge and understanding of the principles of the process of discharge planning will ensure that future healthcare workers are confident and efficient in the process of discharge planning, as well as developing and demonstrating effective communication skills in a safe environment.

CONCLUSION

Discharge planning is a skill of many elements; it is important that the fundamental principles are maintained to ensure a smooth, effective and efficient discharge occurs for the patient.

Effective communications between all involved – healthcare professionals, patients and carers – must occur so that no misunderstanding can happen and cause a delay in discharge. This can be achieved by accurate record keeping in line with professional and legal guidelines. A discharge leader must be identified who needs to take responsibility for the discharge.

While teaching the skill of discharge planning it is important that candidates are up to date with guidelines and procedures within which they need to work.

Resources that may be useful for information to enhance the simulation or for candidates to access following the simulation could include:

- Local Discharge Planning policies
- *Ready to go?* Department of Health (2010)
- The Productive Ward (2009).

Discharge Planning

SIMULATION SCENARIO

This simulation allows candidates to explore the skills required to communicate effectively, especially in difficult circumstances, and to examine the potential problems that can occur when planning a complex discharge.

To ensure effective learning, have a number of candidates as observers who can make notes of what they see. What went well? What didn't go so well? What could have been done differently?

Background Information

Roles

Student nurse, staff nurses, staff nurse in charge, nursing assistants, OT, social worker, physiotherapist, the patient – Mr Jones, Mr Jones' son, consultant – Mr Slater

Patient Circumstances

Mr Jones had a below knee amputation a week ago. He has one son but his wife died recently. She had always been responsible for the shopping, washing, cooking and bill paying. Mr Jones is currently only mobile in a wheelchair and still has clips in his wound.

Mr Jones' notes state:

- He already has a social worker; a message was left for them to contact the ward the day before
- He has been referred to the occupational therapist
- Physiotherapists have been seeing him but it is not clear what the aims of the treatment are
- There is no mention in the notes whether the son has been contacted to discuss the social situation and no phone number has been given.

Actions

Initially

All nurses are at the nurses' station. Mr Slater arrives on the ward and begins to speak to the student nurse in an authoritative and overbearing manner. He begins to explain that he requires a bed for a patient he has in his clinic and suggests forcefully that Mr Jones has been in hospital far too long and should be discharged that day. Staff nurse one is standing nearby and overhears this situation.

What's Next? Options

- If the student does not involve the staff nurse, Mr Slater will turn his attention to the nurse in charge
- If placated Mr Slater will become more reasonable and ask for the discharge to be looked at and moved forward
- If no reasonable response is given Mr Slater will be dictatorial, demand action in the next hour and storm off leaving his mobile number for regular updates.

Other Information Regarding the Simulation

If the staff nurse uses the phone to find out information, there is a list of telephone numbers on the wall near the desk which has two telephones on it.

Any other team members will carry out instructions given to them by the staff nurse.

Anyone who is contacted by telephone will provide information.

Mr Jones will provide his son's telephone number if anyone asks him.

Responses from Telephone Calls if Made

BOX 20.1 – TELEPHONE RESPONSES

Social Worker

States that 'meals on wheels' were being used prior to admission. Asks whether further support will now be required, and says that she will come and visit in the ward this afternoon.

(Continued)

(Continued)

Occupational Therapist

States that they will do a washing and dressing assessment on Friday. Can the nurses make sure that he does not have a wash that morning?

Physiotherapist

Apologises that she has not written in, she was on her way back to do this after being called urgently away earlier on. She predicts that once Mr Jones has a prosthetic limb fitted he will be able to mobilise short distances only.

Son

States that he will be able to do shopping but works full-time and cannot offer much more support. He is worried that his father will not be able to cope at home.

Points for Consideration

- How does the student react under pressure from the doctor?
- Do either of the staff nurses intervene and take control of the situation?
- Is the staff nurse aware of the discharge plan?
- How does the staff nurse placate the doctor, if at all?
- Does the staff nurse check the notes for information?
- Who does the staff nurse contact to develop the plan of discharge?
- Is any new information discovered then recorded?
- Does anyone speak with Mr Jones?
- Do any other members of the nursing staff help out?
- When should a discharge plan start?

REFERENCES

Benner, P. (1984) *From Novice to Expert: Excellence and Power in Clinical Nursing Practice.* Boston, MA: Addison-Wesley.

Bloom, B.S. (1956) *Taxonomy of Educational Objectives, The Classification of Educational Goals – Handbook I, Cognitive Domain.* New York: McKay.

Carroll, A. and Dowling, M. (2007) 'Discharge planning: communication, education and patient participation', *British Journal of Nursing*, 16 (14): 882–6.

Chandler, L., Wyatt, M. and Roberts, I. (2008) *Passing the Baton: – A Practical Guide to Effective Discharge Planning.* Available on: http://www.wales.nhs.uk/sitesplus/829/page/36467 [accessed 25 May 2011].

Chartered Society of Physiotherapists (2010) *Code of Professional Values and Behaviour.* London: CSP. Available on: http://www.csp.org.uk/uploads/documents/csp_code_pilot_nov_2010.pdf

Covey, S. (2006) *The 8th Habit.* London: Simon and Schuster.

Department of Health (DH) (2003) *Discharge from Hospital: Pathway, Process and Practice.* London: DH.

Department of Health (DH) (2004) *Achieving Timely Simple Discharge from Hospital: A Toolkit for the Multidisciplinary Team.* London: DH.

Department of Health (DH) (2009) *The Productive Ward: Releasing Time to Care.* London: National Nursing Research Unit.

Department of Health (DH) (2010) *Ready to Go? Planning the Discharge and the Transfer of Patients from Hospital and Intermediate Care.* London: The Stationery Office.

Foust, J.B. (2007) 'Discharge planning as part of daily nursing practice', *Applied Nursing Research*, 20 (2): 72–7.

Gallagher, A.G., Ritter, E.M., Champion, H., Higgins, G., Fried, M.P., Moses, G., Smith, C.D. and Satava, R.M. (2005) 'Virtual reality simulation for the operating room: proficiency-based training as a paradigm shift in surgical skills training', *Annals of Surgery*, 241 (2): 364–72.

NHS Institute of Innovation and Improvement (2011) *Rapid Impact Assessment of the Productive Ward: Releasing the Time to Care.* London: DH. Available on: http://www.institute.nhs.uk/images//documents/Quality_and_value/productiveseries/Rapid%20Impact%20Assessment%20full%20report%20FINAL.pdf [accessed 19 October 2011].

Nursing and Midwifery Council (2008) *The Code: Standards of Conduct, Performance and Ethics for Nurses and Midwives.* London: NMC.

Productive Series: NHS Institute of Innovation and Improvement (2009) Available on: http://www.institute.nhs.uk/quality_and_value/productivity_series/the_productive_series.html [accessed 19 October 2011].

Rennie, I. (2009) 'Exploring approaches to clinical skills development in nurse education', *Nursing Times*, 105 (3): 20–2.

Royal College of Nursing (2010) *Discharge Planning: A Summary of the Department of Health's Guidance Ready to Go? Planning the Discharge and the Transfer of Patients from Hospital and Intermediate Care.* Harrow: RCN Publishing. Available on: http://emergencynurse.rcnpublishing.co.uk/shared/media/pdfs/discharge.pdf [accessed 26 January 2011].

Salisbury NHS Trust: *Effective Discharge Planning.* Available on: http://www.salisbury.nhs.uk/AboutUs/FreedomOfInformation/PrevFOI/Documents/FOI_355_Q10_Effective_Discharge_Planning.doc [accessed 26 January 2011].

Shepperd, S., McClaran, J., Philips, C.O., Lannin, N.A., Clemson, L.M., McClusky, A., Cameron, I.D. and Barras, S.L. (2010) 'Discharge planning from hospital to home', *Cochrane Database of Systematic Reviews 2010*, Issue 1, Art.No.: CD000313. DOI:10.1002/14651858.CD000313.pub3.

21

DOCUMENTATION

Bernie St Aubyn and Amanda Andrews

Aims

The aims of this chapter are to highlight the problem of poor record keeping by professional practitioners and to provide resources that look at the skills required to write acceptable records. The chapter also aims to explore, through simulation, how poor records could be dealt with in a court setting.

Objectives

The chapter objectives are to:

- Discuss the common features of poor and good record keeping
- Explore the underlying principles which contribute to poor record keeping
- Experience trying to defend records through simulation, in a court setting.

INTRODUCTION TO THE SKILL AND EXPLANATION OF ITS IMPORTANCE AND A RELEVANT DEFINITION OF THE SKILL

Record keeping skills are essential in order to produce court-proof health records. The Data Protection Act 1998 defines a health record as:

Consisting of information about the physical or mental health or condition of an identifiable individual made by or on behalf of a health professional in connection with the care of that individual. (1998: 1)

The key principles of good record keeping include:

- Legibility
- Signed and attributable to a practitioner (for example, to include their name and delegation)
- Dated and timed
- Chronological and contemporaneous
- Accurate and unambiguous
- Factual and relevant
- Comprehensive and include all relevant documentation (NMC, 2009).

Clinical records are the most basic of clinical tools, yet they are often accorded low priority, are poorly maintained and not readily available (Pullen and Loudon, 2006). Records do not simply support patient care, they are essential to it. Record keeping is a non-negotiable clinical skill (Nursing and Midwifery Council (NMC), 2009) that all registered practitioners must be competent at. By maintaining effective records staff are demonstrating their professional accountability and fulfilling their legal and professional duty of care (Central and North West London NHS Trust, 2007). Records are kept by the authorities for seven years or in the case of children until their 25th birthday (Limitations Act 1990).

BACKGROUND TO THE SKILL: WHY? WHEN? RELEVANCE TO HEALTHCARE PRACTICE?

This section discusses why accurate documentation is important, when it is used and its relationship and relevance to healthcare practice.

Substandard record keeping features frequently within allegations in a high number of 'fitness for practice' cases involving both doctors and nurses. In the nursing profession it is one of the top five reasons for nurses being removed from the register or incurring sanctions. In the medical profession the total number of cases with problematic record keeping allegations investigated by the General Medical Council (GMC) in 2009–10 was 508 (GMC, 2011). These include investigations relating to serious concerns and those complaints which were not appropriate for the GMC to investigate in the first instance, but required feedback from the doctors' employer to ensure there were no wider concerns about their fitness to practice. Poor records are often reflective of poor practice and practitioners need to be mindful that this link is often highlighted in court procedures to the detriment of the practitioner. Practitioners are bound by their individual codes of conduct to maintain accurate and factual records. The General Medical Council explicitly states that doctors must:

Keep clear, accurate and legible records, reporting the relevant clinical findings, the decisions made and any drugs prescribed or other investigations or treatments. (2006: 3)

The Nursing and Midwifery Council (NMC) Code for nurses (2008) also clearly states the importance of keeping clear and accurate records. Both of these professional bodies refer to the need for the records to be contemporaneous and legible.

Apart from deliberate acts of record falsification, there are also a number of areas of poor record keeping that could potentially have serious consequences for the patient, healthcare practitioner and the organisation. For example, the omission of a signature on a drug administration record could lead to the dosage being repeated, with the attendant potential risk of side effects for the patient. The healthcare practitioner in such a case might be brought before a local disciplinary hearing. A less serious example may be the failure of a practitioner to date and sign changes in a patient's records. Although this may not have serious consequences for the patient, it could be evidence not only of poor record keeping but also of poor standards of care provision. The use of abbreviations in records that are not readily understood may lead to confusion and a lack of continuity of care for the patient (Quantum Development, 2005).

In an ideal world no healthcare practitioner should need to go to court. The requirement to maintain high standards of record keeping in healthcare professions should serve as a preventative measure. In reality the standard of record keeping in the health service in general is poor and has been criticised by public bodies and official enquiries into deficiencies of care. The Audit Commission's Report (*Setting the Records Straight*, 1995) examined a wide range of issues relating to the management of health records and to the contents of case note folders. It found that the standard of record keeping in NHS hospitals in England was poor and strongly recommended that corrective action be taken. The Audit Commission (1995) identified a tendency for practitioners to treat records as personal rather than corporate assets. There was also noted a lack of coordination between paper and electronic strategies, and practitioners struggled with the need to maintain confidentiality while legitimately freeing up information (Audit Commission, 1995).

Has there been any improvement in the intervening 15 years? Lord Laming's report (*A Progress Report on the Protection of Children in England Following The Death of Baby P*, 2009) stipulates the importance of recording and storing information correctly to reduce the risk of harm. The National Confidential Enquiry into Patient Outcomes and Death report *Caring to the End* (NCEPOD, 2009: 30) states that 'better systems of handover and better documentation must be established to improve patient care'.

Healthcare documentation remains the most tangible evidence of a professional's practice and the means by which it may be judged. The approach to records adopted by the courts is that if it is not recorded then it has not been done.

Court decisions are reached on the quality of the evidence presented to them. Documentation is the practitioner's main defence if assessments or decisions are ever scrutinised. Poor record keeping means that organisations are unable to defend themselves in cases of litigation, as it is this documentation that is examined in court. In many cases of litigation, the claimant can win compensation amounting to thousands of pounds because documentation was not up to acceptable standards. Moreover, healthcare professionals are frequently struck off professional registers for poor record keeping and increasingly held to account for their record keeping, resulting in litigious action against them and/or their employers.

The purpose of completing records is to facilitate communication between healthcare professionals and clients (Twomey and Cummins, 2010). However, anecdotally, healthcare students report that they are not sure what to write, so they tend to copy phrases already written by the trained staff. This practice tends to compound the existing poor quality of records, with a general downward decline in standards as practitioners learn from others' ignorance and inadequate practices.

The skill of keeping good records is an integral part of professional practice because it is an essential part of good patient care. Protection from litigation is not the sole reason for good records, they also provide a chronology which can substantiate that events, conversations, advice and referrals have happened.

They also help to protect the welfare of patients by ensuring high standards of practice and continuity of care. Failure to maintain adequate health records affects not only the practice of the individual but potentially that of their colleagues by possibly causing them to act in such a way as to harm a patient. This could ultimately lead to a charge of professional misconduct (Lynch, 2009). Patient care is generally provided by a multi-professional team and the documentation provides an essential method of communicating between practitioners. Records also play a part in the documentation of risk management by alerting fellow professionals to potential problems and safety issues (Lynch, 2009).

The format of the documents used by health professionals does not always encourage healthcare professionals to complete records correctly. Records tend to require the recording of any *tasks* carried out but omit to document the underpinning quality of care involved in completing the task. Furthermore, less tangible interventions such as listening, teaching and patient advocacy, which are important elements of healthcare provision, tend to be totally ignored in the recording process.

The use of generic documentation in the form of care plans have been found not to be specific enough for individual patients or specialities and are, therefore, perceived to provide little value or add to quality of care (O'Connell et al., 2000). Lack of time is frequently cited by professionals as a reason for the poor completion of documentation (Hardy et al., 2000; Friberg et al., 2005). Sometimes practitioners prioritise the 'doing' of the care above the 'recording' of the care and, culturally, the hands-on caring is considered more worthy. Record keeping, however, should be viewed as an integral part of the healthcare process. There is a tendency to think that the verbal communication at the change of a shift is effective, but this fails to acknowledge the legal supposition that the care not recorded is considered not done.

The impact of the professionalism and confidence of the practitioner in their record keeping ability is also worthy of note. Hardy et al. (2000) discuss how those professionals who lacked confidence in their record keeping skills tended to produce poor records. The belief that their records were not of a high enough standard to be formally reported to others limited their ability to write quality notes. This backs up the notion that record keeping is a skill that is not taught consistently during training and that students' learn from the practice of qualified staff while on placements.

When considering the content of records, ambiguity and repetition need to be considered. Research suggests that most nurses report documentation to be repetitive and a desire to reduce duplication leads to poor notes being completed (Owen, 2005). As documentation is not standardised throughout all healthcare institutions, the ambiguous language used in different settings on different documentation has led to professionals not recording their findings formally.

Electronic record keeping is becoming integral to healthcare with technological solutions being rolled out throughout the NHS. Professionals, therefore, need to be aware of the implications of poor electronic record keeping. The principles of good recording keeping apply whether paper records are being completed or electronic ones being inputted. It has been reported that electronic record keeping is underused by many healthcare professionals who prefer the 'freestyle' method that written documentation allows rather than the formatted and pre-programmed phrases generated by the computer software programmes (Law et al., 2010). Twomey and Cummins (2010) add a note of caution in relation to electronic record keeping, stressing that professionals need to follow local guidance to avoid breaches in confidentiality and errors in information when writing, storing and accessing electronically held records. An improvement in the standard of record keeping needs to be addressed in healthcare to ensure theses errors do not occur.

Poor quality record keeping seems to be common practice. The National Confidential Enquiry into Patient Outcome and Death (2009) revisited common themes from reports written over the past 10 years and one of their key findings was that poor documentation remains commonplace. In summary they found that this hinders effective communication between team members at all levels. The reasons for this may partly lie with the low priority accorded to medical records and/or because national attempts at standardisation are often defeated by the sheer complexity of patient care.

EXAMPLES OF GOOD PRACTICE AND CURRENT UNDERSTANDING AND THEORY

The NHS complaints procedure is responsible for collating and handling complaints made by patients about all aspects of the NHS. Manoj (2009) discusses the issue of how the NHS deals with complaints and draws attention to the fact that at the root of most complaints lie failures of healthcare professionals to communicate effectively; in addition, within many cases record keeping is cited as an element of this. There are a number of examples of good practice in improving record keeping and these should be showcased; the main theme for these improvements tends towards standardisation of records and the productive use of audit to monitor and evaluate.

Sheffield Teaching Hospital NHS Foundation Trust in 2005 and 2006 used an audit to review and then report their resulting recommendations on the quality of record keeping. An electronic pro forma was used as the audit tool and inpatient wards were asked to audit 10 sets of notes. The overall aim was to identify adherence to the Trust's record keeping standards and then develop action plans for future practice. Findings significant to record keeping identified that, although a high standard of compliance was in operation, in 2005 90 per cent of entries were dated, this rose to 95 per cent in 2006 and timed entries rose from 85 to 90 per cent over the same period.

This example of good practice was achieved through the consistent approach of the dedicated project team but also the in-house education and training that was provided and the 'awareness raising' that such a project can generate. It is envisaged by the hospital that in the future the audit tool will be used to examine the quality of the whole records system (Griffiths et al., 2007).

As previously discussed, one of the areas which impact on poor record keeping is the lack of standardisation of documentation and the increasing move towards electronic record keeping is adding urgency to this need. Pullen and Loudon (2006) report that, as the pressure to improve the quality of hospital care increases so does the focus on the structure and content of the clinical records being completed on patients. The Health Informatics Unit (HIU) of the Royal College of Physicians (RCP) in 2007 developed generic standards for all entries into medical notes.

It is envisaged by the RCP that standards for record keeping will allow for improvement in the quality of information we use to judge clinical outcomes by creating a robust framework for the gathering of data generated through the day-to-day delivery of clinical care. An audit tool was devised to monitor the implementation of these standards to determine impact upon the quality of patient record keeping as an outcome of this project.

A joint report produced by the RCP and the Audit Commission was published in 2009 and focused on both improving clinical records and clinical coding. This report had a number of conclusions but, specific to the implementation of the RCP standards, it concurred that the Implementation of the 12 generic medical record keeping standards would improve the order and content of the medical notes, particularly assisting the efficiency of clinical coding and identification of transfers (RCP and Audit Commission, 2009).

POINTS TO NOTE

THINGS TO CONSIDER WHEN TEACHING OR PERFORMING THIS SKILL

Many health professionals say that they have never been taught formally how to record. It is unsurprising then that more than two-thirds of practitioners report inconsistencies in their report writing. Most say they have learned on the job, and 61 per cent say that reading other workers' files has been a significant influence

(O'Rourke, 2009). Policies on recording are not considered particularly helpful – general statements on the requirement to be accurate, relevant, concise and complete are meaningless without practical examples.

Kelly et al. (2008) conducted a study to assess whether students achieved better understanding with the implementation of skills videos within skills teaching sessions. Overall the findings supported the use of videos for teaching clinical skills but in conjunction with lecturer demonstration, not as a replacement – thus supporting a blended approach. Student dissatisfaction was noted in relation to not being able to 'question' the video and this endorsed the findings of Thiele (2003) that students have a preference for an 'expert' being present to question (Kelly et al., 2008). Salmon (2006) identifies the increasing need to move away from 'factory' education, whether that is class-based or distance learning, to a customised method of learning.

The pressures at all levels of education in this country are all-encompassing and institutions of learning are aiming to reduce costs while improving quality and increasing student numbers (Salmon, 2002). The challenge presented in the literature is to devise alternative modes of delivery which move away from the costly lecturer-centred approach to ones which reduce contact time but not at the expense of the quality of the programme (Glen, 2005).

CONCLUSION

In an ideal world no healthcare practitioner should have to go to court. High standards of record keeping should serve as a preventative measure. As discussed above, poor records may result in nurses having to give evidence in either a criminal or civil case. Appearing in court as a witness can be a very daunting and stressful experience, when a practitioner is being cross-examined by a lawyer in the witness box of a Coroner's Court about their records.

Introduction

Simulation provides an opportunity for learners to observe and/or participate in a court room scenario in a safe and protected environment. There is an opportunity through simulation to experience how much easier it is to rebut allegations when supported by well-written, factual, court-proof records.

Learning Objectives

After the simulation the student will be able to:

- Discuss the feelings and emotions associated with such an experience
- Demonstrate and practise the skills required to produce 'court-proof' records
- Recognise poor practice and actively promote good record keeping practice in clinical settings.

SIMULATION SCENARIO

Resources

- If possible – a court room setting to include a witness box. A desk and chair would suffice
- A copy of the patient scenario
- Records – a set of good notes and poor notes recording an episode of care prior to the patient's death
- A prepared statement which the practitioner as a witness will be questioned about
- A clerk to the court to swear in the witness
- Someone to question the witness
- A coroner or judge to keep the proceedings in order
- Videoing equipment to facilitate class-based feedback
- The time for each simulation will be approximately 20 minutes per witness.

Scenario

A patient in the care of the healthcare professional (HCP) has died unexpectedly and this has led to the death being investigated. The notes have been sealed and removed from the setting where the patient was being cared for (for example, hospital, nursing home, community clinic, and patient's home environment). The HCPs involved have been called to appear as witnesses in the Court to answer questions about their care of the patient.

Prior to appearing in the witness box – the HCP will prepare a statement from the notes, a copy of which will have been provided by the court. All witnesses and interested parties have access to the notes, including family members. The HCP is sworn into the witness box and questioned on the care delivered to the patient. The only records available for the HCP to refer to are the notes recorded at the time of the care episode. The HCP experiences trying to give evidence about the care and treatment delivered, under oath, when the only evidence of this care is poorly recorded. The HCP then has the opportunity to give evidence using good records.

Roles of Participants

Witness

The witness/practitioner will be required to familiarise themselves with the scenario and write a statement based on the notes provided. After being sworn-in they will answer questions to the best of their ability from their statement, remembering that they are under oath.

Questioner

The questioner will put relevant questions to the witness to clarify the information included in their statement.

Judge in Charge of the Court Proceedings

The judge will keep order and add to the gravitas of the proceedings.

'Swearing-in' Officer

This officer will be required to facilitate the practitioner in taking the oath or affirmation with appropriate sincerity and solemnity.

Areas for Discussion

Students will be able to compare and contrast the two sets of notes and see for themselves how much easier it is to rebut allegations using the 'good' notes in a legal setting. Students will also be able to recognise and discuss how the behaviour of the barrister is different as a direct result of the quality of the notes.

Points for Consideration

Ensure the environment is safe and allows students to feel able to make mistakes without undue ridicule and destructive criticism. This simulation should promote students' confidence and help them adopt a positive approach with constructive feedback.

REFERENCES

Audit Commission (1995) *Setting the Records Straight*. Abingdon: Audit Commission Publications.

Central and North West London Mental Health NHS Trust (2007) *Record Keeping Policy*. CNWL NHS Foundation Trust.

Data Protection Act (1998) Available on: http://www.ico.gov.uk/for_organisations/data_protection.aspx [accessed 4 April 2011].

Friberg F., Bergh A. and Lepp, M. (2005) 'In search of details of patient teaching in nursing documentation – an analysis of patient records in a medical ward in Sweden', *Journal of Clinical Nursing*, 12: 1550–8.

General Medical Council (2006) *Good Medical Practice*. London: GMC.

General Medical Council (2011) Available on: www.gmc-uk.org/education/education_news/9717.asp [accessed: 4 April 2011].

Glen, S. (2005) 'E-learning in nursing education: lessons learnt?', *Nurse Education Today*, 25: 415–417.

Griffiths, P., Debbage, S. and Smith, A. (2007) 'A comprehensive audit of nursing record keeping practice', *British Journal of Nursing*, 16 (21): 1324–1327.

Hardy, M., Payne S. and Coleman, P. (2000) '"Scraps": hidden nursing information and its influence on the delivery of care', *Journal of Advanced Nursing*, 32 (1): 346–50.

Health Informatics Unit (2007) *Generic Standards*. Available on: www.rcplondon.ac.uk/rcp/clinical-standards/hiu [accessed: 4 April 2011].

Kelly, M., Lyng, C., McGrath, M. and Cannon, G. (2008) 'A multi-method study to determine the effectiveness of, and student attitudes to, online instructional videos for teaching clinical nursing skills', *Nurse Education Toda*, 29: 292–300.

Law, L., Akroyd, K. and Burke, L. (2010) 'Improving nurse documentation and record keeping in stoma care', *British Journal of Nursing*, 19 (21): 1328–32.

Laming's Report (2009) *The Victoria Climbie Inquiry Report.* London: House of Commons Health Committee.

Limitations Act (1990) Available on: www.legislation.gov.uk/ [accessed 5 April 2011].

Lynch (2009) *Health Records in Court.* Oxford: Radcliffe Publishing.

Manoj, G.K. (2009) 'Complaints procedures in the NHS: are they fair and valid?', *Clinical Governance Journal*, 14 (3): 183–8.

National Confidential Enquiry into Patient Outcome and Death (2009) *Caring to the End.* Available on: www.ncepod.org.uk/2009dah.htm [accessed: 4 April 2011].

Nursing and Midwifery Council (2009) *Record Keeping: Guidance for Nurses and Midwives.* London: NMC.

Nursing and Midwifery Council (2008) *The Code. Standards of Conduct, Performance and Ethics for Nurses and Midwives.* London: NMC.

O'Connell, B., Myers, H., Twigg, D. and Entriken, F. (2000) 'Documenting and communicating patient care: are nursing care plans redundant?', *International Journal of Nursing Practice,* 6: 276–80.

O'Rourke, L. (2009) *Practitioners Demand More Guidance and Training in Record keeping* http://www.communitycare.co.uk/Articles/16/04/2009/111259/Practitioners-demand-more-guidance-and-training-in-record-keeping.htm

Owen, K. (2005) 'Documentation in nursing practice', *Nursing Standard*, 19 (32): 48–9.

Pullen, I. and Loudon, J. (2006) 'Improving standards in clinical record-keeping', *Advances in Psychiatric* Treatment, 12: 280–6.

Quantum Development (2005) *Documentation and Record Keeping: How Might they Look in Court?* Quantum Development.

Salmon, G. (2006) *Etivities the Key to Active Online Learning.* London: Routledge Falmer.

Thiele, J. (2003) 'Learning patterns of online students', *Journal of Nursing Education*, 42: 364–6.

Twomey, J. and Cummins, A. (2010) 'Good record keeping', *World of Irish Nursing and Midwifery*, 18 (3): 38–9.

INDEX

Added to a page number 'f' denotes a figure and 't' denotes a table.